Heartmates®

Heartmates®

A Guide for the Spouse and Family of the Heart Patient

THIRD EDITION

Rachael Freed

Fairview Press
Minneapolis

Published by Fairview Press, 2450 Riverside Avenue, Minneapolis, Minnesota 55454. Fairview Press is a division of Fairview Health Services, a community-focused health system affiliated with the University of Minnesota and providing a complete range of services, from the prevention of illness and injury to care for the most complex medical conditions. For a free current catalog of Fairview Press titles, please call toll-free 1-800-544-8207. Or visit our Web site at www.fairviewpress.org.

Library of Congress Cataloging-in-Publication Data
Freed, Rachael.
 Heartmates : a guide for the spouse and family of the heart patient /
Rachael Freed.-- 3rd ed.
    p. cm.
Includes bibliographical references and index.
 ISBN-13: 978-1-57749-121-7; ISBN-10: 1-57749-121-1 (trade pbk. : alk. paper)
 1. Myocardial infarction--Patients--Family relationships. 2. Wives.
 I. Title.
RC685.I6 F69 2002
616.1'23706--dc21

                              2002007884

First edition: 1987
Second edition: 1994
Third edition: 2002

Printed in the United States of America

Interior by Dorie McClelland, Spring Book Design (www.springbookdesign.com)
Cover by Laurie Ingram Design (www.laurieingramdesign.com)
Cover image from an original painting by Igor Levashov, courtesy Winters Fine Art,
        Carmel, California

Disclaimer
This publication is designed to provide accurate and authoritative information in regard to the subject matter covered. It is sold with the understanding that the publisher is not engaged in the provision or practice of medical, nursing, or professional healthcare advice or services in any jurisdiction. If medical advice or other professional assistance is required, the services of a qualified and competent professional should be sought. Fairview Press is not responsible or liable, directly or indirectly, for any form of damages whatsoever resulting from the use (or misuse) of information contained in or implied by these documents.

For wounded families
everywhere
and especially for my own children,
Sidney and Deborah, and for theirs

Contents

Foreword

Fantasies and nightmares produce more unresolved fear than reality. Reality, faced in isolation, can be a nightmare. The reality of a heart attack is unclear because of the way it distorts and fragments the living patterns of a family. Even when the medical staff members suggest that it is a mild heart attack, the family must deal with the distress of unanswered and unanswerable questions. What is the likelihood of death? What will be the extent of disability? Fragments of information from diverse sources cause confusion and despair.

Ms. Freed's useful book, written for those with a spouse who has experienced a cardiac event, will be of great consolation to many. It is a guide to living as a tourist in the harsh, overpowering world of the hospital. It will be as close a companion as any tour book. It is a guide for providing home care for patients recovering from cardiac disease. It is a guide to the perplexing inner emotional experience of living through a heart attack with a spouse. Finally, it is a guide to the intimate handling of that most delicate of heart patients, the marriage.

Heartmates brings help on many levels simultaneously. First and foremost, it is a handbook offering guidance for help in dealing with the hospital and medical staff, with feelings, the family, and marital intimacy. It offers suggestions for diet and coping with lifestyle changes, and it lists resource centers where information is available. There are many brief case examples from the experiences of other cardiac spouses. Finally, interwoven with wonderful delicacy is the story of the author's experience with her husband's two heart attacks and successful bypass surgery. These personal samples are used to illustrate what is too ambiguous to describe.

While the bright light of technological advance in medicine illuminates disease processes, improves survival rates, and reduces the disabling components of serious illness, such as coronary artery disease, the human despair at the center of the experience remains hidden in darkness. The families of heart patients are subject to massive, long-term, often unacknowledged distress. The process leaves the family brittle and lacking resilience.

Case example: Several years ago the Swenson family was referred to me because Bill, age thirteen, the second of five children, had been arrested for vandalizing cars in their upper-middle-class neighborhood. It was not until the third family therapy interview that we discovered that the father, age forty-eight, had suffered a coronary one year previously.

It was no accident we were not told because the family was under the father's strict orders not to speak of his heart attack. In his words, it had been a "mild" heart attack and "could have no possible effect" on the family. Over his protestations, his wife and children described their concern about their husband and father. They were angry that he remained seriously overweight and continued his heavy smoking. The mother said she had not had a full night's sleep since his heart attack, and every time he became upset with the children's fighting, she was fearful it would precipitate another attack.

The father was very upset with me for encouraging his family to talk about their experiences. "It has nothing to do with my son's problems," he repeated emphatically. Yet the family's relief at being able to talk openly was obvious. The tough, taciturn thirteen-year-old vandal told freely about his fears that his father might die. Mr. Swenson refused to bring his family back for another interview. Six months later, the family doctor who had referred them told me that Bill had become a starter on the hockey team, and was back on the honor roll.

This case review gives an example of some less obvious side effects of coronary artery disease. *Heartmates* would have been invaluable to Mrs. Swenson in providing a support for her reality, which was at odds with her husband's. Her reality included her own anxiety symptoms, the distress she could see in their children, and her fantasies about what would happen if he died. His reality included only his doctor's suggestion that it was a mild heart attack and that he could resume his normal work schedule. He had no idea what his wife and children were experiencing, and his denial of death was ludicrous.

Coronary artery disease can be a catastrophic and/or chronic illness, causing problems for the whole family. Health, both physical and psychological, is a function of a family's morale, the family's heart. The clinical tools for helping families under stress have evolved in the mental health professions but have not been integrated into the medical world. Books like this one will educate the families of patients so that they can be more aware of the implications that serious illness in a family member has for them.

As families come to understand the way they are affected by illness, it may lead to changes in the way medical practitioners view the experience of illness. If illness is placed in the context of family living patterns rather than in the simpler individual context, then families can be treated so that patterns of family living do not have a detrimental effect on a member who is ill. Instead, the patterns of family living can be guided so as to enhance recovery for both the patient and the family.

David V. Keith, MD
Director of Family Therapy and
Associate Professor in Psychiatry
State University of New York Health Science Center
Syracuse, New York

Preface to the Third Edition

Heartmates was first published in 1987. Revising it provides the opportunity to appreciate progress and to examine what still needs to be accomplished for cardiac spouses and families.

Healthcare professionals have embraced concepts outlined in *Heartmates* and its related resources, expanding their definition of who their patient is. Whether a person is given a cardiac diagnosis, has a cardiac procedure, or has a heart attack, the event involves the patient *and* his family. The lives of all family members are changed forever by a cardiac event. Healthcare professionals are beginning to treat the whole cardiac family.

Today, family systems and grief theory incorporate the term "vicarious victims of trauma." The phrase legitimizes the issues and needs of cardiac families experiencing an unexpected and life-changing cardiac event.

Most cardiac rehabilitation programs generally include the principles and practices found in *Heartmates* as a routine educational component. Professionals report great satisfaction in using these principles to assist cardiac spouses with their unique and universal needs. Nurses, social workers, and chaplains have welcomed the resource, utilizing it as the foundation of cardiac family educational programs in hospitals and clinics all across North America. And *Heartmates* is available in French and German.

Privileged to travel throughout the United States, Canada, and Israel, I have trained cardiac professionals and addressed cardiac couples. I have heard remarkable stories about the challenges cardiac families have encountered and triumphed over. Newspaper and journal articles, as well as radio and television interviews, have clarified and validated some of the issues cardiac families face.

Of the many cardiac couples I have addressed, only once has a patient or spouse asked about sex in relation to cardiac recovery. This is one of the indications that work on behalf of heartmates is not done. Communication concerns and renewed physical intimacy remain fundamental issues for many people, but they are still difficult to approach.

Understanding that family support and emotional factors play a significant role in the recovery of the heart patient and cardiac family, Marion Laboratories commissioned a series of educational videotapes based on *Heartmates*. These tapes, given to 5,000 hospitals as a public service, provide widespread recognition of the serious crises sustained by cardiac families. A University of Nebraska Medical School study indicates that the video programs aid the heartmate's recovery.

Canada adopted *Heartmates* for its cardiac families with support from Nordic Laboratories. Every Canadian clinic and hospital has the video series in French or English. Nordic Laboratories also provided hospitals *The Cardiac Family Recovery Program Training Manual for Administrators and Facilitators* to prepare professionals to lead programs and classes for cardiac families. They gave physicians multiple copies of the book *Heartmates* to provide to their patient's families. *Heartmates* was endorsed by the Canadian Cardiovascular Society and the Canadian Association of Cardiac Rehabilitation in 1994. Literally hundreds of thousands of families worldwide, isolated and unprepared before *Heartmates* and the Heartmates organization, now emerge from acute shock equipped with skills and understanding.

Since 1994, the Heartmates Web site has assisted heartmates in finding support and reducing isolation <www.heartmates.com>. Literally thousands visit the site monthly for information and inspiration. Heartmates post their stories and questions, as well as respond to other heartmates, on the site's "Interactive Connections" page. I am grateful for the miracle of cyberspace, which gives heartmates the opportunity to find others in similar circumstances throughout the world.

The most recent development is the Heartmates Foundation. It is dedicated to addressing the needs of heartmates worldwide. You can visit it at the "Foundation" page on the Heartmates Web site.

Many heartmates have written that *Heartmates* gives their spirits a needed boost, that the book helps them feel more understood and less alone. Their messages have helped to enrich this new and revised edition. Their letters and e-mails encourage me to continue the effort to bring the Heartmates' vision to fruition, so that heartmates everywhere will be recognized and supported.

May we continue to heal our wounds, adapt to our new, ever-changing family realities, and rebuild our heartmate relationships. May *Heartmates* guide your journey. Mark milestones, grieve losses, and celebrate family each precious day of your life.

Rachael Freed
Minneapolis
September, 2002

Acknowledgments

There are many people who have contributed to my growth and in some way have made this book possible: those I have worked with as colleagues and clients, those I have known personally, and those who have taught me through their writing. I am indebted to all of them. I am especially grateful to:

The cardiac spouses who trusted me with their stories, their pain, their indomitable strength, and their recovery.

Psychosynthesis, its principles and practitioners—it was within that framework that I discovered my sense of purpose.

Elisabeth Kübler-Ross, for her courage to cut a professional path that I could walk on and expand.

Gareth Esersky, my first editor, for believing in the book, guiding me to find "my voice," and giving *Heartmates* elegance.

Denise Silvestro, my second editor, for encouraging me to write for the male cardiac spouse, and for her navigation of the first revised edition.

Tim Larson, my editor for this third edition, for challenging me to deepen and refine the concepts crucial for heartmates' recovery.

Arlen R. Holter, MD, and his staff, for their help reaching male heartmates for my research.

My personal mentors: Harry Sloan, for bringing me to psychosynthesis; Rene Schwartz, who held me as I searched for my truth; Ann Stefanson, who witnessed me finding my *self;* Rabbi Joseph Edelheit, who inspired my return to Judaism; and to Al-Anon, the spiritual program that teaches me self-care and compassionate, detached love of others every day.

My friends, who held me as a cardiac spouse when I most needed it and continue to support me as a woman, which I always need.

My daughter, Debbie Stillman, who assisted in the preparation and writing of an earlier edition . . . for her help and her love.

Introduction

As the spouse (or family member, partner, or loving friend) of a survivor of heart disease, you are part of a growing segment in our culture. You are a heartmate!

About 1.5 million people have heart attacks annually in the United States. Most survive, but heart disease continues unabated. It is our largest disabler and killer. Procedures and surgeries number more than one million every year. As medical miracles and pharmaceutical discoveries revolutionize the treatment of heart disease, survival rates substantially increase . . . and the number of heartmates grows.

Unlike widows, for whom there are behavioral role models, traditional guides for mourning, and respect for the time necessary to grieve and adapt to a major life change, heartmates have no assistance. Heartmates stand alone. Without recognition that cardiac families experience a crisis (are vicarious victims of trauma) even when the patient survives, there can be no help. And no one, professional or friend, can know what specific changes you will encounter as a heartmate; yet, unexpected and permanent change is your reality.

This book was written to provide you with the necessary properties for healing: understanding, support, guidance, and community. This book combines and interweaves practical information, psychological support, and emotional guidance.

Each heartmate is unique, and every cardiac situation is different. This book includes suggestions, tips, and tools, but it does not propose a specific cure for living with the realities of heart disease. What works for one person or couple may not be effective for others. Experiment with the suggestions that feel right for you, and mold them to fit your personal needs and situation. Take what you like and leave the rest.

I have shared my personal story throughout this book to demonstrate how my experience as a heartmate, confronting uncertainty at every stage of recovery, has changed me permanently. (It didn't mean an end to all that was good in my life; nor did it mean an end to unexpected change, or having to relearn the lessons of living with uncertainty, or understanding that I can't control everything.) Personal sharing in the form of "telling my story" has been a healing gift for me.

I am grateful for being entrusted with the lives, concerns, and hopes of many heartmates over the years. I have included some composites of them in this book. Their stories will touch you and inspire you as you journey through this book and your recovery.

And now for some practical details so you can use this book in ways that work for you. A book of more than 300 pages can be overwhelming when you're in a crisis. There is no one right way to use this book. Each reader approaches it from a unique situation and a different point in recovery.

The index should make the content easily accessible. Look through the index first, and then read the topics, usually only a few pages, that meet your needs at the moment.

The book is arranged chronologically, beginning at the hospital and followed by aspects of early recovery. Because of the ongoing nature of heart disease, the plateaus, those periods of maintenance with little change, and setbacks that complicate recovery, you may want to reread the early chapters often, even if you are a longtime veteran of the cardiac experience.

The book leads you from the simple to the complex, from more obvious changes to deeper issues and questions. Themes in later chapters include loss and grief and the healing of relationships with yourself, your mate, your family, and God or your higher power. These issues, fundamental to the quality of our lives, are often the last to be recognized and confronted.

The special needs of the male heartmate are addressed in chapter 7, "Frogs Don't Turn into Princes, but Men Become Heartmates." It is common knowledge that heart disease is the number one killer of men. It is also the number one killer of women fifty-five years and older. About half of those who die each year from heart attacks, and more than one-third of those who have angioplasty procedures, are women. Most heartmates and *Heartmates* readers are women. Chapter 7 briefly expresses the key ideas of the book to address the needs of the growing number of male heartmates.

I think it is important to take a moment to address gender and language: after considering the use of "he/she," I chose to use the traditional "he" when referring to the patient and "she" when discussing the heartmate, for ease in reading. I hope that none of my readers will be alienated or offended.

And, finally, the challenge of the cardiac crisis and journey is facing the reality of your unique situation. At each crossroads along the way, your task is to adapt to change by letting go of what's been lost and developing new perspectives and patterns of action. Finding a "new normal" for yourself and your family that includes heart disease but is not the only focus of your attention will enhance the quality of your life. I hope that you will rely on *Heartmates* as a guidebook for your journey.

May *Heartmates* support you, so you will know that you are not alone. Be strengthened by reading the experiences of others who have struggled with issues similar to your own. They stand with you as you live the difficulties and opportunities of being a heartmate.

1

At the Hospital

*M*y heart racing, I park and run through the darkness toward the double doors marked "Emergency." Where is my husband? The ambulance he arrived in stands empty and there is no sign of him. Only an hour ago we were safely curled up in bed, watching TV and comparing notes on the details of our day. His sudden chest pain and an urgent call to 911 have led me to this door, where I stop, take a deep breath, and realize I don't know what to do.

Once inside, I am jolted by the glare of artificial light, medicinal smells, and an operator's strident voice repeatedly paging doctors. I need to get my bearings, gather my composure, and figure out a plan. But I'm frantic, not knowing whether my mate had a heart attack or is even alive.

I approach the registration desk and am directed to Admitting. A woman behind a computer says to be seated, she will call me. The minutes tick by. I try to keep from screaming at her to hurry up. Doesn't she know this is an emergency? Finally she begins the ritual list of questions, establishing identity, financial responsibility, and the nature of the complaint. I search my mind for my husband's social security number and my wallet for insurance information. I can't believe I'm wasting time doing this when I should be with him. When she's finished, I'm motioned back to the waiting room to resume my vigil.

After an hour, I am told that he is being taken to Coronary Care. I ride with him on the elevator, but when we reach the fifth floor, I'm waved away to wait in the family lounge. I'm not sure what's happening. It seems certain that my husband had a heart attack, but how sick is he? When can I see him? Where is the doctor? Should I stay all night or go home to be with our children and try to get some sleep? How can I possibly sleep? If I leave, will he die?

My body is numb. My mind races a million miles an hour with questions coming so fast and furious that one begins where the last one leaves off. I'm tempted to escape this nightmare, but I don't know how. Instead, I brace myself and walk into the coronary unit. Rules are posted at the nurses' station. Visitors are allowed ten minutes each hour, only one person at a time. My eyes are riveted on a half-dozen monitors, each silently displaying ongoing lines that are images of the patients' heartbeats. On one, the green line is zigzagging uncontrollably in an ominous pattern. What if it's his? What should I do? I tell myself to take it easy; I don't even know how the machine works.

The nurse calmly informs me that my husband is resting comfortably and that I can see him for just a few minutes. Everything is quiet and controlled here, the sounds absorbed by carpeting. I imitate the nurse's measured tone, lowering my voice before entering his room.

Now, after two excruciating hours, I stand at my husband's bedside. I don't know what to say. He's all wired up. There's an oxygen tube in his nose and an intravenous line dripping liquid into his wrist. He is attached to a machine that gives a digital readout of his pulse; it is equipped with a miniature version of the screen at the nurse's desk. Again I stare at the critical green line that mysteriously makes its way from left to right, reappearing again and again.

He says he knows he had a heart attack but isn't in any pain. He asks me to take care of some arrangements at the office and jokes about canceling his breakfast date since he obviously won't be there. His ashen skin and frightened eyes belie his businesslike manner and his humor. I'm not sure how to act, whether I should show how worried I am. Before I've had a chance to sort out my feelings, the nurse signals that my time is up. I lean over to kiss him, careful not to disturb the lifesaving equipment.

On my way out, I stop at the desk for reassurance that my husband will be okay if I leave. The nurse says it's fine to call anytime, day or night. I find my car in the lot and drive home, where I collapse onto our bed and sleep fitfully until dawn.

Whether your introduction to being a cardiac spouse started with your mate's heart attack, a medical procedure, or surgery, *your* crisis began as all do, suddenly and without warning. While heart disease develops over a long period of time, a cardiac crisis happens in an instant. You might have noticed gradual signs, such as your spouse's shortness of breath or a pallor that was unlike his familiar ruddy complexion. But nothing prepared you for the terrifying split-second when you witnessed his heart attack. Nor was there anything to ready you for a seemingly routine checkup that indicated the immediate need for an angiogram, angioplasty, or bypass surgery. At that moment, you were catapulted into a new and frightening reality. With no time to absorb what had happened and no way to know what was ahead, you were propelled into action and forced to deal with a life-and-death crisis.

In many ways, a cardiac crisis is similar to other life-threatening emergencies. Cardiac spouses, however, share the unique experience of being in a crisis precipitated by *someone else's illness.* Your mate is in crisis too, but the experience is not the same. You suddenly find yourself in a situation entirely beyond your control that threatens *your* security and will change *your* future. Unless you have medical training, you are faced with a foreign vocabulary of medical terms you can barely pronounce, let alone understand.[1] You may have to decipher this technical information in order to make decisions with far-reaching consequences on behalf of your mate. And to top it all off, the one person on whom you often rely is totally unavailable. Instead of operating as part of a team, you must deal with this all on your own.

In a crisis, the initial reaction is often numbness. Cardiac spouses describe a sense of being removed from reality, as if they are lost in a dense fog. One spouse described her astonishment at the difference between her experience in the hospital and the larger world:

> *I found myself in a very specialized environment . . . where quiet efficiency was the order of the day. When I emerged from the hospital, I was surprised to see that the world was still there—buses were running, people were laughing and talking, and life was going on as usual.*

During the first few days, you may have trouble concentrating, making decisions, and carrying on conversations with relatives and friends. These are typical reactions. The body shuts down in response to shock to prevent itself from being overwhelmed. It serves as a protective shield, masking the intensity of feelings, allowing you to continue functioning. This is usually a temporary reaction that quickly passes.

> During the first days of a cardiac crisis, it's wise to preserve your energy as best you can. Address only those tasks and decisions that absolutely cannot wait.

Living in Limbo

Once the numbness wears off, you will probably become fearful. It is natural to associate a heart attack with death, despite medical evidence to the contrary. Even though angioplasty, bypass surgery, and newer procedures have impressive track records, they inevitably evoke fear and anxiety.

Anxiety often manifests itself physically. During these first days, while you wait for conclusive information about your mate's condition, you may feel like a tightly wound spring, ready to snap at the slightest provocation. Other symptoms include loss of appetite, trembling, shallow breathing, or insomnia. One spouse I talked with noticed his arm ached, and then realized he had been constantly clenching his fist. Another developed a nervous habit of biting her lip. Fear makes some people withdraw, paralyzes others, and causes still others to become overactive, aimlessly pacing the corridors of the hospital or chattering incessantly.

If your partner requires surgery, those hours of waiting can be the most difficult of all. While it may help to have close friends and family around for support or distraction, ultimately you are alone with your fears. Thoughts about the outcome of surgery bring up a set of survival questions that take your breath away: Will he be in that small percentage that don't make it through surgery? Will his heart beat on its own after being disconnected from the heart-lung machine? Will he breathe when they remove the respirator? Will he get pneumonia? How long will the new arteries work, or will they just collapse? The surgeon's words, "We were successful; all vital signs are stable," offer only partial relief.

Seeing my husband lying in the intensive care unit was dramatically different from anything I could have imagined. There were neither windows nor clocks in the cubicle, and time felt indefinitely suspended. His hold on life seemed so tenuous. Every part of him was hooked up to something. He was at the center of a whirlwind of activity. Skilled, efficient nurses moved swiftly in and out, executing complex life-sustaining procedures. I knew that morphine protected him from pain, but he was restless and straining against the respirator. His hand and arm, still chilled from surgery, felt like a stranger's. All the while the regular rhythm of the monitor reassured me with its beep . . . beep . . . beep. I returned to the waiting room totally shaken by what I had seen. He couldn't even breathe on his own. How would he ever be healthy and whole again?

Once the initial crisis passes, your worries continue, intensified by the unknown. While you are relieved that your mate has survived, new questions arise: What are the details of his condition, and what is the long-term prognosis? Will he have constant pain? Will he be dependent on medication? Is he going to be an invalid? Will he be able to work, to travel, to lead an active and fulfilling life? What are the chances of another heart attack?

Most of us have a hard time coping with the unknown. Learning to live with uncertainty is one of the heartmate's greatest challenges. Knowing that your mate is in competent, professional hands can alleviate fear. While it's essential to get all the information and medical guidance you need, it's also important to recognize that even the most gifted physicians cannot foretell the future. The best they can provide are percentages for recovery. Medicine, for all its awesome accomplishments, is still a limited science.

Your anxiety will diminish as you become more secure about your mate's survival and as the repercussions of his illness become clear. In some hospitals, trained social workers and chaplains are available to help you through this traumatic time.

> Voice your concerns. Acknowledging your fears to someone, or even aloud to yourself, can reduce their power.

Ruth, a soft-spoken woman in her early fifties, drove her husband forty miles to the hospital emergency room. After his examination, she was told to follow him and his entourage of medical staff to the intensive care unit. At the big double doors, she was stopped and told to wait outside. No one explained what was happening.

Ruth sat alone in the silent corridor for close to an hour. During that time she considered every possibility. She didn't think she would ever see Ralph alive again. She reviewed the highlights of their thirty years together, thinking about what he meant to her and how much she would miss him. She recalled their dreams and tried to imagine pursuing them alone. She even planned his funeral, picturing herself there with their three sons.

The doors of the intensive care unit swung open and a nurse emerged. Ruth, lost in her own thoughts, was startled. The nurse told her that Ralph was doing well and that she could come in to see him. She burst into tears of joy and relief.

The hour spent waiting was a turning point in her life. She had begun to prepare herself emotionally for the loss of her husband, confronting squarely the possibility of living as a widow. Ruth rose to go to her husband feeling strengthened and confident in her ability to cope with whatever would be their new reality.

Fears intensify in the midst of crisis. The urgency of the situation makes it almost impossible to keep things in perspective. Lack of information increases dread, and we imagine worst-case scenarios. We are accustomed to having physicians give us authoritative answers, so any ambiguity can be interpreted as bad news. Some people naturally cope with the unknown by adopting a positive attitude—they know survival is a given. Others are more likely to envision the worst. When told that 98 percent of those who have bypass surgery survive, they automatically count themselves with the remaining 2 percent.

Anxiety in the face of the unknown is a normal and appropriate response, as long as it doesn't impair your ability to function.

> Exercise cautious optimism. Combine a positive outlook with a realistic appreciation for the gravity of the situation. That way you can hope for the best and still be prepared to cope with contingencies.

Making Yourself at Home

As you struggle with your fear about your mate's survival and recovery, you need to deal simultaneously with a new and strange environment. For all intents and purposes, you have taken up residence at the hospital. You may spend periods of time at home or at work, but your mind and your heart are on the cardiac unit. Trading the familiarity of home and work routines for the alien atmosphere of the hospital further distorts your reality and can make you feel disoriented. Your schedule is completely out of kilter, and your sense of time is governed by hospital routine: rotating shifts, the return of the latest test results, and the doctor's rounds.

How do you handle the hospital? First, you must recognize what part the hospital plays in your emotional experience. On the one hand, it's a relief to see your spouse safely attended by professionals who can, in many instances, save and prolong his life. On the other hand, the hospital system was not created to address your needs. The physical layout, efficient pace, and antiseptic environment is designed for critical care and maximum productivity. Its primary purpose is to accommodate the patients and medical staff.

You, too, however, have needs, basic human needs that arise in crisis, including a need for understanding and comfort. In order to feel comfortable, you must first understand the lay of the land. It's frustrating to find yourself on the Employee Only elevator en route to a supply room.

> Find your way around. Know the location of the lounge, the telephone, the gift shop, the coffee shop, and the chapel. Doing so will contribute to a semblance of order.

Once you get your bearings, the next step is to understand the inner workings of the system. This is what I call "cracking the code." A hospital is a unique world, with its own language, customs, and culture. Your aim is to effectively maneuver and negotiate on behalf of yourself and your spouse. This necessitates learning the procedures, vocabulary, and chain of command.

At times you may feel frustrated or in the way. Everyone else is rushing around doing an important job, while you hurry up and wait for visiting hours, for a few minutes with the doctor, for test results, for rehabilitation meetings. In some ways your needs seem at cross-purposes with the running of the hospital. You trust your physicians' competence more when you see how busy they are. But because of their pressing schedules, they make their rounds before you can get there in the morning or during the half-hour you leave to get a cup of coffee. And when you finally catch up with one, you forget an important question you meant to ask. You admire the nurses' ability to handle so many things at once. But their cheery, upbeat appearances and their exhausting routines make you hesitant to bother them with your questions. After a while, it all feels like a conspiracy to keep you in the dark.

There is nothing you can do to change the doctors' rounds or the nursing staff's style, but *you have every right to ask them questions*. If there never seems to be an appropriate time to do so, set up a specific time to discuss your concerns. Speak with your cardiologist and nursing staff directly. Instead of anxiously waiting for your doctor's appearance, call the office to make a formal appointment or find out when he or she will be on hospital premises.

Heartmates often perceive the hospital staff as a lifeline, but this can make you feel dependent on them and cause you to be especially careful in your relationships with them. You worry about asking too many questions or being labeled pushy or demanding. You might be hesitant to arrange for the privacy you know will make your mate more comfortable. You may be afraid of making a wrong move, inadvertently doing something to antagonize the doctor or nurses and thus jeopardize your partner's care.

Whether or not it's justified, it doesn't take long to get the idea that if you're "good" and wait patiently without making waves, your mate will receive first-class service from the staff. Many cardiac spouses are reluctant to express their opinions, thinking that their input will be construed as interference, criticism, or doubt. One heartmate never came to the hospital without bringing candy for the nurses. Another always prefaced her questions with an apology, fearing the nurses would think she was stupid or wasting their time. Another felt hesitant to tell the nurses that her mate was someone of great age and dignity and that it would be more respectful to call him "Mister" than to use his first name.

Early in my husband's hospitalization, I wrestled with the conflict between my desire to be seen as a "cooperative spouse" and my need to participate in his care.

In an educational session with the coronary care nurse, we were shown a chart of "mets," the units of energy expended in each physical activity. It covered the period from the heart attack through six weeks of recovery, listing the graduated activities that would ultimately lead to resuming a normal life.

The following day, my husband was moved to a cardiac recovery unit. A nurse appeared and informed him that he had bathroom privileges. I knew she was wrong. According to the mets chart, bathroom privileges were several days off. Although it wasn't ten yards away, I reacted as if my mate was being encouraged to sprint around a track or take an extra base on an infield single. As much as I wanted him back on his feet, part of me wished he could permanently remain in coronary care and never again do anything that took any mets at all. Why tempt fate? Better he should do nothing more active than breathe, and live.

I didn't want the stigma of "trouble," but I was determined that he not get out of bed until the chart permitted. I found the charge nurse, waited until he was free, and told him that my husband did not have bathroom privileges and wouldn't for several days. He checked the chart, agreed, and thanked me for letting him know.

After this clarification my fear subsided, but only for a moment. In its place a new dread appeared: if this error could be made, so could others. I knew I'd better stay alert and be prepared to speak up in case a more dangerous mistake occurred. If it were necessary, I'd move in and stand guard twenty-four hours a day.

Combating Helplessness

It's natural to feel helpless when you are caught up in events beyond your control. In some ways you truly are helpless. Nothing you can do will turn back the clock. You can neither change nor ignore the fact that your spouse has heart disease. There's no way to reverse the risk factors and lifestyle choices that contributed to this crisis. And unless you are medically trained, you are incapable of providing the technical care that's required. It's important to acknowledge these realities, but it's equally valuable to recognize your power.

Most of us endow physicians with too much power. In a crisis, we're apt to expect physicians to work miracles. Terrified, we expect them to have all the answers and never make mistakes. Once we make the doctors omnipotent, it's difficult to have appropriate expectations of them.

By giving up so much power to your doctor, you diminish your own. If you have a question or idea, you may stifle it, thinking, "I've never been to medical school," or, "If the doctor thought it was necessary, he'd have recommended it." What you don't take into account is that *no physician knows everything*. Regardless of how smart or dedicated a doctor is, no one can keep up with every new development in a field.

Your doctor is the medical expert, but you know more about your mate than anyone else does. And no one cares as much about this recovery as the two of you. Sharing your knowledge can be crucial in planning a successful recovery program with the staff. Studies show that spousal support is the most influential element, "the heart," in the recovery of heart patients.

You can increase your power and self-respect by educating yourself about heart disease. The more you know, the more you will be able to contribute to your spouse's recovery. Christina, an avid reader, came across a ten-year study of a medication thought to reduce cholesterol rates. Her husband, Paul, had undergone an angioplasty procedure, and she wondered if the new medication might be a significant addition to his diet and exercise program during recovery. Christina clipped the article and showed it to their doctor, who followed up and prescribed the medication.

Sometimes we withhold valuable information because we feel intimidated or shy. Your intimate relationship with your spouse makes it especially important for you to speak up. Stuart, a quiet and intuitive man, felt terribly uneasy sitting beside his dozing wife, Kim, the first night following her bypass surgery. Despite assurances that Kim was in stable condition, he was seized with a sense of foreboding. Something was wrong, and while he couldn't put his finger on it, the feeling was impossible to dismiss. When a nurse passed, Stuart asked her to check Kim, who indeed was developing postsurgical complications. Within minutes, emergency measures were taken and a potential disaster prevented.

Information is another factor in counteracting helplessness. It is your need, your right, and your responsibility to have access to all the available data.[2] Ask your nurse or hospital social worker for a copy of your patients' bill of rights. People in Minnesota, for example, are protected by state law. Of the twenty-six sections in the Minnesota bill of rights, four are especially pertinent to cardiac family members:

- Patients have the right to be treated by the staff with courtesy and respect for their individuality.

- Patients have the right to be given complete and current information concerning their diagnoses, treatment alternatives, risks, likely results, and prognoses by their physicians in language they can be expected to understand.
- Patients (including a family member) have the right to participate in the planning of their healthcare.
- Patients have the right to a prompt and reasonable response to their questions and requests.

HEARTMATES® HOSPITAL QUESTIONS

Here is a guide for asking questions and gathering information. Read over the items. Note the questions that concern you the most and add new ones as you go along.

Heart Attack
- What is a heart attack?
- What does "heart damage" mean?
- How long does recovery take?
- Will my spouse need a procedure, surgery?
- What causes a heart attack?

Medication
- What is the medication supposed to do?
- What are its potential side effects?
- How long does the drug need to be taken?
- How frequently is it taken?
- What happens if a dose is missed?
- What is the generic name of the drug?
- What are the reasons for changes in medication?
- What should we do if he can't remember having taken his pills?
- How do the prescribed medications interact with each other?

Surgery and Procedures
- What happens during the angioplasty procedure?
- What happens during bypass surgery?
- When is a procedure or surgery indicated?
- What are the advantages and risks?
- Who is best qualified to do the surgery?
- Where can we get a second opinion?
- How soon should the procedure or surgery be done?
- How long does it take to recover from angioplasty or bypass surgery?
- What is the desired outcome?

Recovery
- When will my mate be able to come home?
- What lifestyle changes should be made?
- What kinds of stress should be avoided?
- Will he have to change his job or retire early?
- What kind of emotional reactions should I expect from my spouse? Will he be depressed or angry? For how long?
- Will we be able to resume sexual activity? When? Are there any dangers involved in having intercourse?
- How often should we schedule appointments with the doctor?
- Will the hospital provide any ongoing support?
- Whom should I call to answer my questions?

> Your list of questions is undoubtedly lengthy and will change daily. Put them in writing to help you remember them, to mark the significance of your concerns, and to bolster your confidence.

Once you have compiled a list of questions, decide who can best respond. Some questions should be directed to your family doctor or your cardiologist. Other questions require the expertise of the nursing staff, the exercise physiologist, the nutritionist, or a veteran cardiac spouse.

You are absolutely entitled to all the information you need. If the answers you receive are too vague—such as, "Oh, that's nothing to worry about" (easy for you to say), or, "Time will take care of that" (how much time?)—it's your right to ask for clarification.

Sometimes it may be important to consider why you're not getting the answers you need. An unsatisfactory answer may be precipitated by an unclear question; you may need to be more specific. Recognize, too, that some of your questions may not have definitive answers. Differences in family, religious, or ethnic background between you and the professional staff also may make communication more complex or difficult.

Some doctors are comfortable answering questions and are sensitive to your feelings and concerns. Others are defensive, unresponsive, and noncommittal. They may brush off your questions for a number of reasons, including time pressures, lack of communication skills, and discomfort discussing issues that are personal or painful.

Ideally, your doctor is someone whose medical expertise you trust and with whom you are personally comfortable. But, as in any relationship, no one is perfect, and you may need to accept that this fact applies to your doctor as well. Your doctor may be a respected expert in cardiology but have limited experience in a variety of surgical procedures. He or she may enjoy the best medical reputation in town but have a bedside manner that leaves something to be desired. Feeling angry or ignored, you may forget that your doctor is on your side. Appreciation and a "thank you" may soften the tenor of your questions and the doctor's responses.

What matters is knowing what will make you feel most secure. Out of loyalty to your doctor, you may feel that you should unconditionally accept his or her judgments. In truth, your only obligation is to pursue a course of treatment that will facilitate your mate's recovery, provide for your peace of mind, and honor the human dignity of you both. If you want a second opinion, get one. If the two conflict, get a third opinion. If you and your mate are ill at ease with your doctor, look for another.

The Communication Bridge

When someone you love is hurting, it's normal to want to help. During the hospital stay your contribution may seem superfluous. From the moment your mate arrives, professionals and technology take over and you are relegated to the background. You would do anything in the world to help, but it feels as if there's nothing you can do.

Find things to do that have a utilitarian function. You will simultaneously do something that is needed and something that will make you feel like you're part of the team, rather than a helpless interloper.

Some of the most important tasks you can perform involve communication. By promoting communication you fulfill a much needed bridging function between your partner and the world. You can, for example, serve as a bridge between the busy professional staff and your spouse, who may be unable to talk immediately following a procedure or surgery. You can communicate with your mate, helping bridge the gap between reality and the haze of shock and medication. You are also the logical person to assume the role of communicator for family, friends, and people at work, who want and need to know about your spouse's condition and progress. (For more about this important and fatiguing function, see "Directing Communications" in chapter 4, pages 97 to 99.)

Right after surgery, your spouse is totally vulnerable. The respirator and throat tubes make verbal communication impossible. He has no way to make his simplest needs known. Bring your spouse something to write on so he can communicate his needs.

> Help your mate express himself after surgery by providing a Magic Slate (the children's writing toy), an erasable marker board, or a notebook and a pen.

Some ways you can anticipate your partner's needs go beyond verbal communication. Moistening dry lips, moving a sheet that's pulling on tubes, or readjusting a pillow, for example, sends a nonverbal message of your caring. Other needs may require the expertise of the nurse. Your partner may be anxious about a machine that has changed the rhythm of its "beep," and you can ask the nurse to explain.

The first days following surgery are distinguished by a drug-induced haze that protects your spouse from pain, but may also cause him alternately to doze, be easily startled, be out of touch with reality, or say bizarre things. One woman reported that her husband thought he was being experimented on in a concentration camp. Another man admonished his family to hurry to the midnight buffet on the promenade deck of their cruise ship.

Add powerful medication to an absence of windows or clocks in the cardiac care unit, and the already strange environment can be overwhelming. Simply telling the patient the time and whether it is day or night can provide an important reality check. Letting him know how long he's been there may furnish significant direction for his return to the world of life and the living.

Checking medication is another way to act as a communication bridge. You can actively participate in your mate's care by learning the names, dosages, and purposes of drugs being administered and sharing this information with him. He will feel some control over his own care if he can monitor his medications for dosage accuracy and take them on time. Both of you will feel more secure if you understand how the medications work.

Your presence is significant to your mate because it is a symbol of stability and reality at a time of extreme confusion and vulnerability. With no other frame of reference available to him, you are your mate's connection to his earthly roots, his home, his family, his recovery, his life.

Caring for Yourself

Being a bridge is both a gift to your mate and a way to reduce your helplessness. By giving, you increase your power. But it's equally important to be able to receive. In a cardiac crisis, everyone's focus is understandably on the patient. You, too, however, are physically and emotionally vulnerable. Your daily schedule has been disrupted, you are spending most of your waking hours at the hospital, you are deeply affected by your mate's illness, and you are trying to juggle your spouse's needs with the other demands in your life.

Adequate rest and proper nutrition are two things that are often neglected during a crisis, but you can't afford to lower your resistance. It will make you less effective and more susceptible to illness. You must eat regularly and get sufficient sleep. Food from vending machines and the hospital cafeteria can be marginal, so it's a good idea to eat a nutritious breakfast at home. You might also pack a bag lunch and bring healthy snacks to eat in the family lounge. You need to keep your energy and spirits up, and, besides, sharing a snack with other cardiac families in the lounge may be a much needed ice-breaker.

You may feel exhausted from the stress of the situation. Short naps can help to compensate for disturbed or disrupted sleep. Rest when your spouse does.

Even if you are normally sedentary, take a walk at least once a day. Take a break from the confines of the hospital and get some fresh air. Returning to the outside world, even for a short time, can clear your head and replenish your resources.

I can't emphasize enough the importance of support during this crisis situation. You run the risk of becoming depleted or resentful unless you take care of yourself, too. This is an appropriate time to let yourself be taken care of by friends and relatives who are willing to bring food, accompany you on walks, or visit with your spouse so that you can take a break. You need and deserve support. There's no reason to try to do it all alone.

Before You Leave the Hospital

Many hospitals offer cardiac patients and spouses an educational program to provide information about diet, exercise, risk factors, stress, and sexuality. These classes are usually held while your mate is still hospitalized, with the purpose of preparing you to go home.

In order to facilitate this process, let your nurses and doctors know what you need. It's safe to assume that the hospital staff members want to help, that their goal is to promote healing. That doesn't make them mind readers. Tell the staff if you have forgotten a detail from an earlier meeting and would appreciate hearing it again. If you are having trouble concentrating, say so. Be specific about areas of concern, and keep on asking questions until you get the answers. If you feel embarrassed by your lack of knowledge, remember that you are in a totally new situation. These sessions are *for you,* so be sure to take advantage of the information and support.

Later, let the staff know how practical and worthwhile the educational sessions were. Your feedback is bound to benefit cardiac families in the future. And the staff, committed to quality care, will appreciate your perspective.

A good educational and support program will:

- keep educational meetings short (no more than ten to fifteen minutes),
- provide time for each couple to discuss the information during or after each session,
- make a question box available for individuals who are uncomfortable speaking in a group,
- offer at least one meeting for cardiac spouses to identify their most pressing questions and concerns regarding preparations to take their spouses home, and
- provide clear and simple handouts covering the material discussed.

As you and your partner move into the recovery phase, you may want to participate in an educational program that meets regularly. This can be very valuable as you make the transition from the acute crisis into the next stage, which brings its own new issues and concerns.

The hospital experience is only the beginning of a long-term situation heralded by the cardiac crisis. Issues that begin here will follow you home. You will have to learn to deal effectively with the medical community; it's an important part of life with someone who has a chronic condition. A positive way to approach this challenge is to develop an ongoing relationship with your hospital staff members.

Since heart disease is a chronic disease, as yet incurable, this may be your first of many times at the hospital. Nine weeks after my husband's first heart attack, he had another. Sudden changes in his condition brought him back to the hospital two years later, resulting in bypass surgery after an angiogram. Fourteen years later he had a second coronary bypass. Should you need to return to the hospital, you'll feel more at home if you have participated in educational programs and meetings in the interim.

There will continue to be areas over which you have no control. You have neither the power to eradicate your partner's heart disease nor to eliminate its effects on your life. In time, you will adjust more and more to living with uncertainty. But for now, your primary goal, as you anticipate bringing your mate home from the hospital, is to be prepared to support his recovery and yours.

CHAPTER 1 NOTES

1. See glossary for clarification of medical terminology.
2. It's validating to hear other healthcare professionals state what I know from my experience as a cardiac spouse and from my work as a clinical social worker. In his 1997 traveling seminar, "Family Health and Chronic Illness," William J. Doherty, PhD, master teacher, author, and groundbreaking clinician, stressed that when there is a life-threatening diagnosis or an acute event, families usually rally, and they need access to "what's going on." They need information.

2

On the Road to Recovery

The phone hasn't stopped ringing all morning. Everyone wants to know when my husband will be home so they can come over to see him. Soon everything will be back to normal—our lives will be just the same as they were before his heart attack. Driving to the hospital to bring him home, I feel eager and excited. These past days have seemed like forever. I'm grateful that there were no complications, that this nightmare is almost over.

I arrive at the same time as his favorite nurse. Upbeat and professional, she carries a thick packet of papers that she ceremoniously turns over to me. In it are exercise diagrams and schedules, cholesterol tables, and scores of heart-healthy recipes. The nurse gives us one last reminder about avoiding undue stress and checks to make sure we have medications for this afternoon. Finally, she hands me several prescriptions and instructs me to have them filled immediately.

I feel somewhat reassured by her orderliness and efficiency, but I'm a little nervous about taking my husband home. Is he strong enough to wait in the car while I stop at the drugstore, or should I drop him off at home and then go fill the prescriptions? I don't know what to do; my head is full of conflicting details and directions. I'm beginning to feel as though I've accepted a Mission Impossible assignment without fully realizing how difficult and dangerous it might be.

The nurse insists on a wheelchair. She assures me that my husband's fine, that it's hospital policy, but I feel as if I'm taking home an invalid.

The back seat of the car is filled with gifts, books, and six large plants accumulated during his stay. We're finally on our way home, the two of us, surrounded by symbols of life and love from all his well-wishers.

We stop at our neighborhood drugstore, and I rush in to get the pills. It seems to take longer than it should to count out a few pills and label the bottles. I'm shocked at the cost, but quickly write a check and rush back to the car. He looks a little worn. I think about "undue stress" as I drive toward home and decide not to mention how expensive the prescriptions are.

Tears of joy fill my eyes as the kids throw their arms around their dad to welcome him home. They stick around to keep us company while I unpack. I arrange the plants all around the bedroom to attract energies of healing, growth, and life. But with the hospital water pitcher, the medicine bottles, and the pile of new books, it still looks like a sickroom.

By this time my husband says he's tired and is going to take a nap. It's hard for me to imagine how he could be tired from just riding home from the hospital, but I say nothing and leave him to sleep.

I sit down with my packet of recipes and instructions, but I can't concentrate. I'm drained, but too wound up to relax. I feel disappointed that we haven't really talked or celebrated his homecoming. For days we have lived in public view, and I have had to share him with doctors, nurses, and technicians. The logical voice in my head begins to instruct me about what I should be thinking and feeling. "Calm down," it says. "You should lighten up, feel grateful, say a prayer of thanksgiving. Everything will be just as it used to be."

It wasn't. That first day home was only the beginning of the emotional upheaval that followed. Little did I know how much a heart attack had already changed my life.

What happened to me and what is happening to you is this: You have lived through the initial phase of a crisis. You are beginning to adjust to changes that began abruptly and are beyond your control. These changes have already affected you, and they will continue to affect your life in ways that you cannot yet predict. Even homecoming, the anxiously awaited reunion with the family, turns out to be far different from the anticipated "return to normal."

The myth is that everything will be the same as it was. The truth is: *nothing will ever be the same again.*

New Ingredients

Any life crisis brings change on many levels. Early in the cardiac crisis the basic elements of your lifestyle are the most noticeably affected. At a time when you especially need nourishment and rest, you are coping with new dietary programs and disrupted sleep. No aspect of your life is immune to this crisis. Your work schedule, leisure time, and social life have been disrupted and altered. Your primary relationship is in transition. Even your personal goals and dreams, beliefs and values, are undergoing change as a result of your mate's heart disease.

Adopting a heart-healthy diet is a paramount concern for most couples in the early stage of recovery. Before you became a cardiac spouse, you were probably only vaguely aware of diets that may have prevented heart disease. You may have gradually shifted your family away from red meats and toward fish and fibers. A heart-healthy diet is not much different from the general trend toward nutritious eating. But for the cardiac spouse it involves more than wanting to be fashionable or fit. It feels as if it is a matter of life and death. And that puts a lot of pressure on you.

Before my husband's heart attack, our family's diet was primarily Midwestern: meat and potatoes. I salted liberally, and never checked prepared foods for sodium, fat, and cholesterol content. Meals, which were previously a casual affair slipped in between our teenagers' various extracurricular activities, became a major undertaking.

I had to learn to cook all over again. I found myself unhappily spending hours in the kitchen absorbed in recipes, meal planning, and food preparation. It reminded me of being a newlywed, trying to impress my husband with delicious and healthy meals. I experimented with herbs and spices to replace the deadly salt I had been warned against. I searched for recipes that would transform the taste of broiled fish into sirloin steak.

There is general agreement that diet may improve recovery and prolong a heart patient's life, but a new food plan requires time and planning. It can't happen overnight. One extra milligram of salt in your spouse's soup will not cause him to keel over on the spot. You may feel guilty about the eating habits you have taught your family, or you may even believe that your cooking method was a primary cause for your spouse's heart disease. But only in recent years has a correlation between diet and heart disease been seriously considered. Years ago, low-sodium and trans fatty acids were hardly household words. There's no reason to blame yourself; you did the best you could. To cry over whole, not skim, milk is neither productive nor constructive.

Use your new knowledge positively now and in the future. During a time of crisis, when everything is upset and upsetting, you need to make changes gradually.

> Let go of regret over past cooking practices, and focus on what you can do now.

Preparing healthy meals is a way to contribute to your mate's recovery. For many couples, making dietary changes together can be a statement of shared commitment and an opportunity for closeness. While a cardiac diet may seem to lack variety or spice, it offers a potential second chance at life.

A new food plan is a positive signpost on the road to recovery, but it may unfortunately also become a dangerous detour. For some couples, changing eating habits is a source of conflict and stress. It's common for partners to disagree about how significant a factor food is to recovery. Partners can find themselves in disagreement about strict adherence to a food plan when it comes to selecting which foods to eat and which foods to avoid.

Food choices and meal planning can be difficult territory for a cardiac spouse. You want to do everything in your power to help your mate stay on a healthy diet. Your spouse is also an adult, who has the responsibility to choose to eat wisely.

Adjusting to a rigid new diet requires effort and discipline. Most recovering heart patients take a break from the approved list of foods now and then. It's normal to feel concern about your mate's commitment to a healthy diet. But everyone deserves an occasional treat.

Overly critical comments or controlling behavior may reflect your fear of losing your spouse. Arguing about food may also be a way for both of you to indirectly express fear and release anger about your situation.

Suzanne took a three-month leave of absence from her job as a computer programmer in order to care for her husband, Jim, who was recovering from surgery. She devoted herself to cooking delicious, healthy meals and helping Jim stick to his diet. If they were meeting friends for dinner, Suzanne called ahead to check the menu or brought along a separate meal for Jim. One night Jim arrived home with half a dozen chocolate brownies and devoured all six. Bristling with anger, Suzanne blasted him, "Chocolate! You may as well eat poison."

Suzanne's perfect recovery plan was ruined. She didn't want Jim to be deprived of pleasure, especially since it was the first time he had broken his diet since the surgery. But watching him eat six brownies made her realize how terrified she was of losing him.

Monitoring your mate's diet can be a way of trying to maintain control in a situation that is overwhelming and actually beyond your control. In a time of crisis, when the usual ways of expressing love and caring are disrupted, the preparation of food takes on more significance. In most relationships, sharing food connects people emotionally.

Cardiac spouses often report a lack of appreciation for their efforts. Angelina, the cardiac spouse of a proud Italian restaurant proprietor, spent night after night making heart-healthy meals. After years of pasta in cream sauce, she assumed that Carlos found the cardiac fare boring and bland. One day Angelina drove across town to a gourmet grocery to buy special herbs for dinner. All through the meal she waited for Carlos to comment on her chicken rosemary. He ate silently. Finally, she asked him if he liked the meal. His response: "I prefer it plain."

Angelina was crushed. She interpreted Carlos' reaction as a personal rejection of her and her cooking. In fact, his lack of enthusiasm probably had little to do with Angelina or her efforts to please him. More likely it was a statement about his own change in values regarding food, an indication of depression, or a sign of his effort to cope with his new diet. (Many recovering heart patients become disinterested in food, or decide that food is a less important priority in life.)

During this transition, communication is every bit as important as cuisine. There is no diet plan that will assure immortality, no one way to prepare or eat food that is right for a particular couple.

> Talk with each other about food, about dietary changes, and about how to negotiate this ongoing adjustment in your lives.

FOOD ISSUES TO DISCUSS WITH YOUR MATE

Here are several questions about food to prompt discussion with your mate:

- What are our important issues about food?
- How do we each feel about sticking to a food plan?
- Who is responsible for changing and controlling the diet?
- How do we want to handle exceptions to the diet ("cheating")?
- How can we resolve disagreements about food?
- Are we both willing to eat a heart-healthy diet?
- How can we share responsibility for a new food plan?
- How can we best take care of ourselves in relation to food and diet?
- How can we support each other as we re-form our eating habits?

It may be new for you to think seriously about what you eat and how you feed your family, but understanding your beliefs and feelings about food will prove useful. Because diet is a cardiac risk factor, the emotional stress attached to it is high. But we all have to eat, and the cardiac spouse can choose a brand-new, healthy approach to food.[1] You have the opportunity to follow a healthier food plan, one that is more satisfying and nourishing for both of you.

Getting Your Rest

It is essential for you to maintain your own health and well-being so you can support your mate's recovery. While caring for the patient, you may unconsciously place your own needs for sleep and healthy eating second. Cardiac spouses often report that they are too worried or anxious to sleep. Interrupted or fitful sleep is a natural reaction to stress. Once the initial numbness and shock wear off, it is normal to remain on guard and tense. If your whole life changed in an instant, it might happen again at any time. Your entire being responds to the continuing threat of danger. The initial crisis has passed, yet it is difficult to relax and, sometimes, to sleep.

There probably isn't a cardiac spouse anywhere who hasn't awakened abruptly in the middle of the night, ready to dial 911. I spent many nights holding my breath, listening for the sound of breathing, waiting anxiously to see the blanket move gently up and down. It reminded me of being a new mother, always listening for the baby with one ear.

Recovering cardiac patients often sleep fitfully and need naps during the day. This change may be temporary, caused by new medications and the trauma of going through a heart attack or cardiac procedure. Irregular sleep or changes in your mate's sleeping patterns aren't necessarily danger signals or something to be concerned about. Still, it may take some time before you will be able to fall asleep peacefully, confident that your partner is all right.

You may also be worried that lack of sleep will be a setback to recovery. Having been told that rest is an essential part of the healing process may increase your anxiety about your partner's restlessness. *But worry doesn't help.* Although it took many months, I finally stopped asking my morning worry question, "How did you sleep last night?" For me, the report of how many times he had awakened in the night, or of how long he lay tossing and turning, counting and recounting the meager number of hours slept, only served to aggravate my concern. We'd both been awake, and we'd worried together, but it did nothing to improve his sleep or mine.

Eventually, the patient's new sleep patterns will become more routine and less frightening to you. In the meantime, you need to restore and maintain your emotional and physical energy.

> Get all the rest you can. This may mean cutting back on some of your activities or taking the phone off the hook so that you can grab a nap.

A short period of conscious relaxation (see appendix A for an exercise designed to help you relax) can release tense muscles and calm nervous feelings. Deep breathing works wonders when you feel too tense to sleep. Take in a long, deep breath through your nose, and exhale slowly and completely through your mouth until you feel that all the air is out of your lungs. Repeat this five to eight times. Try using these relaxing breath breaks frequently throughout the day to reduce tension, too.

Sleep disturbance often occurs because partners wake each other up. It may be difficult for you to get used to sleeping in the same bed again after hospitalization. Some couples handle the problem by sleeping separately.

> Unless absolutely necessary, I caution against sleeping in separate beds, as it may become a permanent barrier to sleeping together.

Once one of you has moved to a separate bed, it may be difficult to find a reason to return. The time apart may create feelings of shyness or a reluctance to ask for the physical closeness you need.

Give yourselves time to get used to your new reality and you will find that your sleep patterns will be less disrupted. For the sake of your rest and in order to preserve your closeness, talk with your mate about sleep. Remember, you, too, have been through a crisis. It takes rest and care for *your* body and *your* heart to heal.

SLEEPING HINTS

- Give yourself permission to nap during the day.
- Take the phone off the hook when you rest.
- Consider earplugs to protect your sleep from your mate's restlessness.
- Don't rely on medication for sleep or relaxation.
- Let go of your expectations about adequate sleep.
- Don't count the minutes and hours that you sleep; let how you feel be your guide.
- Listen to quiet music before going to bed.
- Drink something warm, soothing, and decaffeinated in the evening.

Working Out Work

During the early weeks of recuperation, no one knows how complete recovery will be. This can be a fearful and frustrating time of uncertainty about your partner's career. Try to remember that 85 percent of surviving heart attack victims are physically able to return to normal activity within three to six months after a cardiac event.

You may be confronted with some changes in your spouse's career or work schedule. Doctors may recommend that your mate reduce his work hours or change jobs to something less physically or psychologically demanding. In some cases, it may be necessary for your spouse to take early retirement. For those in a family-owned business, nothing changes things more quickly than to have the boss suddenly away because of a cardiac problem.[2]

I remember worrying incessantly about whether my husband would be able to go back to work full time. It was excruciating to wait, not knowing if he would be permanently disabled or handicapped by angina. Most of all, I worried about the uncertainty of our future. I felt especially anxious about our financial responsibilities; we still had two adolescents at home. Like most heart attack survivors, he was fortunate to be able to return to his work, at first part time, and as his strength returned, full time.

I have worked with cardiac spouses who were less fortunate. Claudia and Peter, both in their mid-fifties, were told after Peter's bypass surgery that he should change jobs. Selling real estate was too stressful. Before Peter's surgery, Claudia's salary had been supplemental. Her night job as a nurse's aide now became their sole source of income. As they watched their life savings dwindle, their fear and depression intensified.

They sought professional help. Classified as "disabled" by the state, Peter took training in a government rehabilitation program. After one full year of unemployment, Peter found a job. No one addressed what the stigma of being labeled "disabled" meant to him, just as earlier no one had considered the stress he would undergo being unemployed.

Six months later, Claudia became ill and had fibroid tumor surgery. Her strength through the cardiac crisis and the year of Peter's unemployment, her stability as breadwinner and wife, had taken their toll. For a time she became the patient and needed to be cared for.

Whether your spouse retires, changes vocation, or stays with the same job, it's important for you to be involved in making the decisions. You may hesitate to express your opinion because you don't want to add stress. But the stress already exists. Your questions and concerns are probably similar to your mate's.

It is *normal and stressful* for heart patients to be concerned about what recovery really means, asking themselves any number of questions: Will pain prohibit my normal activity? Will reduced cardiac efficiency keep me from working at my regular pace? Will I have to change jobs? Will my partner respect me if I retire or make less money? Will we be able to pay the bills with less income? What kind of sacrifices will we have to make?

Economic pressures are only one aspect of work stress during recovery. Returning to work creates new tensions. Employers may under- or overestimate how long your mate needs to shift gears. Fellow workers may want to discuss your spouse's cardiac experience when your spouse wants to forget that it happened. Or conversely, colleagues may be uncomfortable talking about heart disease and avoid your mate's need to talk.

Discussing all these issues can reduce the burden each of you is carrying alone. Together you may be able to devise a creative plan to cope with the financial distress and the work situation. Two heads are better than one, and being supportive of each other's recovery will yield benefits to both.

Your Career

You may be involved in your own career as well as trying to facilitate your mate's recovery. Your family situation may necessitate making temporary or permanent adjustments in your work schedule or even changing jobs to provide for your family. At the same time it is important that you don't neglect your own career and career needs.

One of the hardest lessons I learned as a cardiac spouse was the importance of going on with my own life. I had to alter my work schedule to account for the changes that were happening in my personal life. At times I was too distraught to give my full attention to my therapy clients. There were days when I felt guilty for being healthy, going off to work, and leaving my husband at home alone. I felt uncomfortable sharing my enthusiasm and sense of accomplishment about work because I thought he might feel envious or anxious about his own career. At other times, work was a refuge, a place where I didn't think about myself and I could focus on someone else. I needed to return to my work because it gave me stability and a sense of normalcy. It also helped to reduce my anxiety about our finances.

Some cardiac spouses sacrifice their own careers because of their mate's heart disease. When Marjorie first came to see me, she complained of boredom. As a young, single parent, she had developed a successful management career and had raised her three children. She recalled her loneliness during those years, but her responsibilities to her children had kept her working hard, and her success was a source of great satisfaction. She considered herself a valuable member of society.

Once her children were grown and her responsibilities reduced, she began to see Phillip, a business colleague. Although he was ten years her senior, they decided to marry. She had the best of both worlds: a stimulating career and a husband who was a close companion and an equal in business.

After four wonderful years together, Phillip had a seriously damaging heart attack. Marjorie decided to retire with him, although she was only fifty-three. Since the onset of heart disease, Phillip and Marjorie have been inseparable. The only time they are apart is once a week, when a friend comes to take him out for lunch. Marjorie misses the stimulation of her job and her old way of life.

Honoring her marriage at the expense of her career, Marjorie has sacrificed an important aspect of her identity and her self-esteem. Now she is looking for something that will give her own life a broader meaning. But a lifestyle change is not so simple. Phillip relies heavily on her for care, attention, and security. She feels responsible for his health and worries about what will happen if there is another emergency and she is gone. She faces the complex situation of regaining her individual life meaning without jeopardizing her commitment to her marriage.

> Coping with career needs and changes can be extremely stressful for both of you. There is no one right answer for any cardiac couple, but it's important to discuss these issues early. Avoiding them won't make them disappear.

In fact, ignoring this topic may become the biggest problem of all. Consider seeking professional counsel if you and your mate cannot talk about work and career issues or reconcile them in mutually satisfactory ways.

Discussion can clarify how each of you is learning to make adjustments and redefine priorities. Brainstorming about work can be practical and productive. Once you can talk, you may discover new options. You may be able to use each other as a reality check. You may even discover that your feelings are similar. Perhaps together you can devise a plan of flexible reentry into the work force.

If you talk about your mutual concerns, this recovery period can also be a time to get reacquainted as a couple, and to begin long-term planning based on your realistic reappraisal of possibilities and new priorities. Sharing your concerns may ease fears, diminish loneliness, and allow you to develop your teamwork skills.

Simple Pleasures

Obviously, your social and leisure activities have been affected by the "cardiac lifestyle." What seemed before like simple decisions—whether to go to a movie or play doubles tennis—become major issues in adjusting to a heart-healthy life. You want to protect your mate's health, but at the same time maintain your friendships and other interests.

When I first met Loreen, a thirty-seven-year-old cardiac spouse, she was trying to cope with changes in her social life. Six weeks after Tony's heart attack, Loreen planned a celebration barbecue for some of their friends. It was a beautiful summer evening. Everyone enjoyed the company, the good food, their new deck, and lovely yard. Loreen felt pleased with her party and grateful that her life, so recently in chaos, was back to normal. She glanced at Tony and found him fast asleep in the lawn chair. It wasn't even dark yet! And what about their guests?

Loreen talked about how she felt that night: lonely, embarrassed, angry, and sad. She also shared her concern about her future. What other lifestyle limitations would she encounter? How would she control her resentment if, at thirty-seven, her social life were to be permanently restricted? Loreen's questions are not hers alone. Many cardiac spouses wonder the same things, especially during the active recovery stage (the first three months after a heart attack or a procedure), as the cardiac patient regains strength through a combination of rest and graduated activity.

It is not unusual for a cardiac patient to nod off occasionally, even when something interesting is happening. You may feel embarrassed or impatient if your mate drifts in and out of conversation or moves at a snail's pace. You may question his motivation or even harbor resentment that he isn't improving more rapidly.

> You may need to alter your expectations of your partner during recovery. The cardiac patient needs time and psychological space to integrate the many changes resulting from heart disease.

There isn't anything you can do to speed up the recovery process. However, there are ways to adapt to it. During this period, you may ask your friends to be flexible in accommodating themselves to your needs. Likely, they will be understanding and tolerant of the situation and grateful to participate in recovery. A rigorous night at the bowling alley may be replaced by a quiet evening watching movies and munching salt-free popcorn at your home or theirs.

Your Personal Active Life
As the weeks go by and your spouse's physical recovery progresses, you may wonder when it's appropriate to return to your hobbies and friendships. At what point is it okay to resume your weekly tennis game, luncheon out with friends, an evening bridge game, volunteer work, the monthly book club meeting, or other activities you were involved in before?

You may feel guilty going out and enjoying yourself when your partner is home in bed. Or you may think that the seriousness of heart disease precludes recreation and fun. Some cardiac spouses are afraid of criticism, worrying that being seen in public "having a good time" when a spouse has suffered a heart attack implies that they are insensitive, uncaring, or selfish. Others just don't feel the old enthusiasm for projects that had been important before all this began.

There is a possibility that your mate sustained substantial heart damage that will permanently restrict his physical activity. You may be a marathon runner, or just a weekend jogger, but your mate may now find it difficult to walk a flight of stairs or get through dinner without being short of breath.

Some cardiac spouses give up their own physical activities to reduce the differences and avoid conflict. Others change their activities temporarily or adjust to match their mates' paces. If you are feeling uncomfortable about exercising when it isn't an option for your partner, be sure to talk about it together. Keep in mind that your choices may be short-term and that your mate's condition will continue to change.

> Assess *your* physical health and emotional well-being before making a final decision about eliminating activities or exercise from your active life.

The decision to resume your own activities is, ultimately, an individual matter. It's very important to be involved in something besides caring for your recovering mate. Time for yourself, whether it's reading a book, exercising, or shopping with a friend, is an important part of this transition. Maintaining interests in other areas of your life is essential for your own needs and to restore a realistic balance to your relationship.

Your Shared Active Life

The cardiac lifestyle doesn't require you to trade in your collective running shoes for canes and bifocals. Set the old bedridden stereotype aside. Every cardiac couple is different when it comes to the level of expectation for social and leisure activities, but you can realistically expect your mate to make gradual progress and to have more energy each week.

Medical trends stress the importance of regular exercise to strengthen the cardiovascular system and the general health of the heart patient. If your spouse participates in a cardiac rehabilitation program, he will get the supervised exercise he needs as well as a support network of fellow patients. Recovery programs usually encourage cardiac spouses to participate.

Exercising together has several benefits. It is another opportunity for closeness and companionship, as well as an opportunity to share an activity you enjoy doing together. Regular exercise is important for your physical health, too. It is an antidote for restless nights, irregular appetite, and general lack of energy.

Adding regular exercise to your routine requires effort, but it will more easily become a part of your schedule if you plan physical activity together three or four times a week. Whether you walk, bike, swim, or exercise more strenuously, what's most important for health is to exercise regularly. Check any new exercise plan with your doctor before you begin.

On the Road Again

For many of us, visiting and vacationing are a natural way of life. Whether we're heading to the shore, the mountains, the family cabin, or the kids' house to witness the grandkids' newest achievements, we like to travel.

When heart disease enters the picture, things change. What were once eagerly anticipated visits and vacations become fraught with fears, concerns, and uncertainty. Though doctors often lift restrictions on travel after the early weeks of recovery, many heart patients experience difficult feelings about traveling.

So do heartmates. Derek, for example, experienced fear: "I'm too scared to go on vacation away from her doctor and hospital." Harriet also felt fear: "His heart attack happened away from home on a business trip. It was so hard there, away from family and friends. I never want to travel again." Shelley had a very different reaction: "My heart is broken. We used to spend a weekend a month driving down to see our grandchildren. It's been four months since his surgery. He refuses to travel and won't even tell me why." Pam shared her guilt and frustration: "We always said that when we got to this age, we would see all the places we dreamed of. I feel so cheated and guilty because I blame him for getting sick, for being so involved in his own health and not even noticing my desire to travel. What can

I do with my get-up-and-go energy? How can I stop resenting him and his heart disease?"

When your normal routines change, whether by choice or circumstances beyond your control, stress increases. Your anxiety button gets pushed, probably because anything out of the ordinary automatically activates the memory of your mate's cardiac event or fear about the possibility of another. Things aren't as certain as they once seemed, and this produces anxiety.

Since that unexpected moment, you have used much of your energy to keep everything orderly and safe. Wanting to travel brings you face to face with a paradox. You want everything to stay under control, safe and secure, unchanged. But by its very nature, travel is a break from routine. A trip can be a wonderful change, offering new sights to see, new people to meet, new experiences to savor, and new learning. It also offers a new set of circumstances that you can't control.

Setting your mind at ease will allow you to enjoy your travel more fully. Everyone experiences some discomfort with the unexpected. Plan ahead, and share the responsibility for planning with your mate to ensure that you have a safe and successful trip.

> You and your partner will have more control if you anticipate your special needs and plan for them *before* you set out for your destination. This is the first step in planning your next trip.

The second step is to do your homework. Visit your local library, talk to a travel agent, or surf the World Wide Web. You might find the following resources helpful in getting the latest information about travel:
- AARP: <www.aarp.org/travel>
- Elderhostel: <www.elderhostel.org>
- Medical Travel: <www.medicaltravel.org>
- Senior Travel: <www.senior.com/travel>
- Society for the Advancement of Travel for the Handicapped: (212) 447-1928

- ThirdAge: <www.thirdage.com/travel>
- Traveling Doctor: <www.traveling-doctor.com>

Use your favorite search engine to discover other sites and contacts—there's always something new in cyberspace. And now it's time to pack!

THE HEARTMATES® PACKING LIST

Your doctor and professional staff can provide answers to many of your questions about travel. Call the office for clarification about travel matters, including:

- Destination. Heart patients may need to avoid high altitudes (such as the Rocky Mountains or Andes) and cities or countries with poor air quality. High altitudes mean a lower oxygen level, and lack of oxygen places greater stress on the heart. Poor air quality requires the heart to work extra hard to get enough oxygen.
- The safety of mixing heart medications with common travel medications for air or sea sickness, stomach upsets, diarrhea, and so on.
- Referral to a physician or health facility in the city or area you plan to visit.
- Obtaining a copy of your mate's most recent cardiogram and history to carry in your wallet or purse. Your doctor's office staff can mail, e-mail, or fax a copy to you.
- Verifying specific cautions your doctor might have for your mate. Clearly state and agree to any limitations before you and your spouse leave home.

The following are some tips to minimize your travel concerns:

- Carry a duplicate set of medications in a separate place for the duration of your trip. Always travel with medications in your carry-on luggage or purse. Keep a complete set of written prescriptions with you as a secondary precaution.

- Travel wisely: Give yourself plenty of time so you reach your flight gate without the stress of rushing. Check luggage through to your final destination. Use curbside check-in whenever possible. Use carts to negotiate long distances in airports and train stations.
- Make a habit of checking emergency medical procedures when you arrive at the hotel, just as you check the fire evacuation plan and exits from your room. If 911 isn't used, familiarize yourself with the procedure to get emergency help.
- If you don't already have one, buy or rent a cell phone, especially for automobile trips, so that access to emergency help is only 911 away. Be sure to provide family members with the cell number and other contact information.
- If you plan to travel outside the country, contact the embassy or consulate there for a list of English-speaking doctors. Phone numbers for embassies and consulates are available through your local library, many travel books, the Web, your travel agent, or a travel service.
- Check with your insurance agent for the availability of emergency or evacuation insurance for foreign travel.

These simple preparations can reduce your fear and enhance your trip, freeing you to experience the excitement, the fun, and the stimulation of travel. When you feel anxious, take a deep breath and remind yourself that you and your mate are okay and well prepared. Have a great time!

Who Are You Now?
A Question of Identity

You can change the way you cook, and you can adjust to coming home earlier on Saturday night. You can exercise regularly, and you can learn to live with less money, and you will still be you. But the changes that cardiac spouses experience go deeper. They affect the very center of your identity.

Identity is often experienced in the roles you play in daily life. People commonly identify themselves according to their responsibilities, by what they do, not who they are. For example, common primary roles are: wife, mother, sister, daughter, friend, lover, coworker, volunteer, and partner. In addition, your identity is dictated by your beliefs about the world. If you say you are an optimist, a "people person," or a devout Christian, you are identifying yourself in another way.

As a cardiac spouse, your roles and your beliefs are in a process of unexpected change. Since the onset of heart disease, when you were first faced with all those new responsibilities, you have assumed new behaviors. Continuing to maintain your regular activities, you have also taken charge of healthy meal planning, medication schedules, visiting hours, and keeping your family intact.

Since a cardiac crisis happens quickly and requires immediate action, it is natural to step into new roles without even noticing you're doing so.[3] But stop here to look; you may be surprised to see that you have taken on one or more of the following roles.

The Head Nurse

- Does your everyday vocabulary include words like angina, edema, stress test, triglycerides?
- Have you become an expert on the side effects of medications?
- Are you constantly adding questions to your list for your next call to the doctor?
- Is it difficult for you to go "off duty" and just relax with your mate?

If these traits sound familiar, you may be wearing the crisp starched cap and white uniform of the head nurse. Although your patient load is light, it really matters. Keeping track of medications and communicating with the doctor may have become your official duties. Although you may have no medical training, you feel fully responsible for your mate's recovery.

It may be reassuring to take on the nurse's role, because the duties are clearly defined. However, it can be exhausting to feel as if your mate's health depends on your constant medical supervision. Even though there are pill bottles everywhere, your home is still your home, not a hospital. You are needed as a helpmate and a partner, not as a nurse.

The Traffic Cop

- Are you constantly on guard for danger?
- Are you regularly pointing everyone in the "right" direction?
- Do you check to see if each medication is taken on time?
- Do you pride yourself on your ability to make fast decisions?
- Are the words "slow down" always on the tip of your tongue?

It is perfectly natural to want to take charge, replace chaos with order. There are schedules to be followed and decisions to be made. It's important to take your responsibilities seriously. Heart disease is no laughing matter. It isn't necessary, however, to acquire the stiff-brimmed hat and dress blues of the traffic cop.

Your well-meaning efforts to keep your mate's recovery on track may have unconsciously embodied an unhealthy authoritarian stance. It's stressful for you to be on duty all the time. And your mate may interpret your concern as control rather than support. Perhaps it's time to turn in your uniform and whistle. Guiding, not directing, traffic will be better for both of you.

The Chef

- Have you purchased more than two new cookbooks in search of heart-healthy recipes?
- Do you feel discouraged when your mate doesn't compliment you on your culinary skills?
- Do you insist on bringing your mate's own meal from home when you are invited to someone's house for dinner?
- Do you spend hours reading nutritional charts?

If creating heart-healthy meals has become your full-time career, you may have slipped into the role of the chef. Constantly seeking healthy, delectable recipes, you hope to aid your mate's recovery and elevate his spirits. Being the chef is a way for you to feel positively involved in improving your mate's health. You probably feel let down, however, if, after slaving away in the kitchen, he doesn't appear to appreciate your efforts.

If you take off your chef's hat and apron, you will be less likely to set yourself up for disappointment. Cardiac patients may temporarily or permanently lose their enthusiasm for food. Your mate's appetite is not a reflection of your culinary ability, of who you are, or of his love.

The Mother

- Do you find yourself wringing your hands, pacing the floor, constantly worrying?
- Do you find yourself talking to your mate in a soothing, pacifying, maternal tone?
- Is all of your attention devoted to your mate's care?
- Are you afraid to leave your mate home alone in case he needs your help?

When someone you love hurts, it is natural to feel protective. But if most of your time is spent coddling and taking care of your mate, you may have unknowingly taken on the role of the mother. Mothers are known for their nonstop worrying and selfless giving. It's one reason why they're always so tired.

Right now it may be necessary to do more than your usual share. But if you have a perpetually worried look on your face, you may be taking on more responsibility than is good for either of you. Treating your spouse like a youngster will only add to his feelings of helplessness. After a while you may begin to resent his demands. Your mate needs your help, but he doesn't need you to be his mother. And you don't need him to be your child.

Coping with Change

As you can see by looking at all the stereotypes described above, much more than your lifestyle has been changed by the cardiac crisis. You may not be aware of how much your roles and identity have changed. Most people find it difficult to be objective about themselves, which can limit recovery and their ability to adapt to changes inherent in dealing with their partners' disease.

The Heartmates Assessment of Change that follows will help you assess the changes in your life. Many cardiac spouses have found it valuable to write their responses in a notebook or *The Heartmates Journal,* a companion volume to this book. Writing clarifies thinking; it's a safe way to express feelings, and it creates a useful reference for the later stages of recovery.

The assessment is organized by major categories of change, such as sleep, diet, and exercise, to help you organize your thoughts. Subcategories follow under each general category to guide your exploration of specific changes. Consider each aspect of the assessment as it relates to your life before and after the cardiac crisis. Once you've completed your assessment, read on to learn how you can use your findings to cope with change.

HEARTMATES® ASSESSMENT OF CHANGE

Sleep
Quantity
Quality
Disturbances
Dreams and nightmares
Frequency of naps

Leisure Activities
Types of involvement
Schedule and hours
Level of commitment
Level of satisfaction
Priority in your life

Diet
Level of appetite
Time spent shopping
Time spent in food preparation
Frequency of eating out
Primary foods
Priority in your life

Financial Responsibilities
Providing income
Budgeting
Allocating funds
Handling banking

Work/Career
Degree of involvement
Schedule and hours
Level of satisfaction
Quality of work

Exercise
Type
Frequency
Quantity
Strenuousness
Regularity

Friends/Social Activities
Differences between you
Frequency
Quality of time spent
Level of satisfaction
Initiating activity

Using Your Assessment to Cope with Change

Once you have an objective sense of the changes that have already occurred, you can begin to understand those with which you are satisfied and where you want to initiate further change. If you notice that you have let an important friendship lapse, for example, invite that person over or plan an outing together. On the other hand, you may be very pleased with the modifications you've made in your diet.

Given the unexpectedness of the cardiac crisis and the pace at which you have functioned during your partner's recovery, it may be a real relief to stop and take stock. The ability to step back and look at the situation, your life, and your weaknesses and strengths is a good sign that you are on the road to recovery.

It may be difficult to go over financial papers, wills, and insurance. Not only is it challenging and time consuming, it forces you to acknowledge mortality. But once you have done it, you may find a sense of peace and empowerment replacing the panic in your chest. Facing your fiscal reality increases your trust in your own resilience and flexibility. The nightmare of having to sell all your possessions will be replaced by a more realistic assessment of your resources and earning skills. If you've always left the finances to your mate, pretending you don't have a head for figures, then assuming more responsibility might increase your confidence in yourself. You might even find that you like doing the family accounting.

Taking an objective look at yourself and your situation is an essential part of coping with change and comprehending what has happened to you. It is equally important to acknowledge your strengths in dealing with the crisis thus far.

> Take time to recognize that you have managed these difficulties to the best of your ability, and that you can adapt to change.

It isn't easy to affirm your strengths. Most of us are more comfortable with criticism than with compliments. We find it difficult to appreciate our positive qualities, although we are acutely aware of our weaknesses. You may even be admonishing yourself with internal dialogue: "I should be more caring and attentive. . . . I should be more worried about him. . . . I shouldn't relax my vigil. . . . I shouldn't feel bad, sad, or mad. . . . I shouldn't have a good time or enjoy myself. . . . I don't deserve to give myself any credit for handling the cardiac crisis well, because I haven't done it perfectly."

No one is perfect. Taking credit for doing your best is an important part of the recovery process. Something that has worked well for many cardiac couples is making a pact to share one thing each day that you appreciate about yourselves. That way a realistic and ongoing assessment of your situation can continue. You will also have something worthwhile to talk about every day.

Continued assessment of the ongoing changes will help you recognize and accept reality and your ability to cope with it. I wish I could tell you that the road to recovery is straight and narrow, but I know that it rarely is. The road sign reads "Uncertainty." Accepting this requires a new belief in your ability to be flexible in order to survive, even thrive, with ever-unfolding, permanent change.

Coming to terms with change and uncertainty can be the most difficult part of aftercare. The road is different for every cardiac spouse.

For some, there may be more potholes and unexpected turns. If you are fortunate, recovery will be a long, lasting journey, and the reality of living your life with someone with heart disease may be accepted as simply part of growing older together.

Chapter 2 Notes

1. One of my favorite cardiac cookbooks is *Craig Claiborne's Gourmet Diet,* written by Craig Claiborne with Pierre Franey (New York: Ballantine Books, 1980). It includes low-sodium and modified-cholesterol recipes. Our family's favorite recipe is "Lemon Chicken, Texas Style." See also the very useful books by Joseph C. Piscatella (Workman Publishing) of the Institute for Fitness and Health: *The Fat Tooth Fat Gram Counter* (1993), *The Fat-Gram Guide to Restaurant Food* (1997), *The Don't Eat Your Heart Out Cookbook* (1994), *Controlling Your Fat Tooth* (1991), and *Choices for a Healthy Heart* (1987).

2. When the owner of a family business has a cardiac crisis, two basic steps need to be implemented: continuity planning and leadership transfer, followed by sharing the plan with everyone involved. Note that there are professionals who work with family businesses in every major city.

3. Dona Wilson, cardiac spouse program facilitator in cardiac rehabilitation in Carson City, Nevada, collected hats designating the stereotypical roles described in this chapter for her support group. After trying on a hat picked from the basket, each spouse reads the description of the matching role. Spouses experience the roles that go with each hat without guilt, and animated discussion follows.

   If you wish to share something useful from your recovery, please write us at: Heartmates, P.O. Box 16202, Minneapolis, MN 55416, or <heartmates@heartmates.com> (e-mail). You can also contact us through the Interactive Connections page of our Web site at: <www.heartmates.com>.

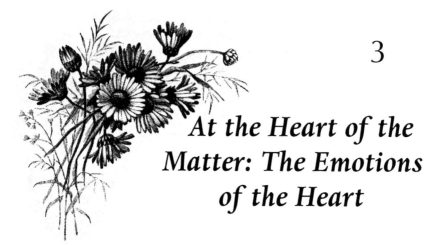

3

At the Heart of the Matter: The Emotions of the Heart

I recently encountered a woman whose husband had just passed his six-month mark. I congratulated her on his recovery. She nodded thanks, but something about her expression made me wonder if she was okay. When I gently asked her how she was doing, she recounted a familiar story.

Ever since her husband's return from the hospital, their marriage had become increasingly stressful. Before his surgery they had been compatible and close. Now they vacillated between bickering and strained silence. Their home, which had always been a haven, now felt like a battleground, and they, like shell-shocked survivors.

Her story reminded me of how difficult a love relationship can be in the first six to twelve months of recovery. At the same time, I recalled that there is much to be thankful for during these months: You can feel grateful beyond measure that your mate has recovered, regained strength, and is back on his feet. The image of him weak and vulnerable in the hospital slowly fades. You might scarcely recall fitful sleep and irregular meals, or the sense of disorientation and helplessness. You have probably acquired enough technical terminology and expertise about medications and diet to run an educational program at the hospital. Your partner has not called a doctor in weeks, maybe even months.

It's a relief to settle back into a regular routine. The new order, incorporating scheduled exercise and dietary changes, is almost second nature. There is less pressure on you to care for a patient, and you have enough time for family, activities, and work. Friends and relatives have returned to their normal lives and don't call or visit as often. Some days you don't even react when you get an unexpected telephone call or hear an ambulance siren.

It's important to recognize and be grateful for your partner's recovery and a return to "normal" living. Celebrate that recovery. It's also crucial to understand that your transition continues. What was normal before bears little or no resemblance to life as you know it today. Some days you will feel great; other days you won't seem able to pull yourself out of the doldrums. Understanding this period of continuing change and striving for balance will help make this transition easier for you.

It's Your Transition and Relationship, Too

You probably consider your partner one of the half-dozen people you are closest to in the world. Before the cardiac crisis, you may have told your mate about things that were important to you. You probably discussed opinions and issues on a regular basis. You may have shared inner secrets, hopes, and dreams. At times, you experienced the satisfaction of physical closeness and sexual intimacy. You felt a connection, partially crafted and honed by years spent living, playing, working, and perhaps raising a family together.

Your relationship with your partner has changed in both obvious and subtle ways. There are a number of issues that make this period especially complicated. The one person you normally count on for support is emotionally out of reach. Ironically, your mate may be around more, but you feel lonelier than ever.[1] Heart patients, as a rule, are engrossed in their physical symptoms. Even when your spouse is physically present, his preoccupation with himself may leave little room for your needs.

Your mate may also demand more of your time or want you nearby just for security. Activities that you used to share, like volunteer work or league sports, may no longer interest your partner or may be limited because of medical restrictions. If your routine keeps you at home with your recovering spouse, the increased proximity may hamper your mobility and freedom. You might even begin to feel smothered, as if you are losing yourself in this entity called heart disease.

The onset of the cardiac crisis caused a major break in your relationship. First, there was the physical separation. You slept at home while your mate, surrounded by medical equipment and strangers, slept in the hospital.

There was a breakdown in communication. The shock of the crisis made you unsure of what to say or how to respond. You got the message that your spouse needed rest and shouldn't experience stress. You hoped your partner wouldn't notice the dark circles under your eyes, a product of stress and sleeplessness. Instead, you were the cheerleader who encouraged his short, slow walk down the hospital corridor. You tried to act cheerful and upbeat when you really felt worried and sad. You held back your tears so that he wouldn't be burdened by your anguish. The more you withheld your feelings, the greater the distance grew between you.

For some couples, there is a carry-over of that emotional distance into the recovery phase and beyond. You may still be as withdrawn as you were when you stood at his hospital bedside. Your communication with each other may be stilted for fear of creating stress or making each other feel worse. You may even believe that your relationship is so fragile that it would disintegrate if you started talking.

You may not be aware of the energy it takes to disguise your feelings from your mate. And, in the long run, you are setting up a mode of communication that inhibits rather than promotes honesty in your marriage. Your partner may wonder what really lies beneath your cheerful countenance or resent your apparent confidence when he is feeling so scared. Besides, *he needs to be needed now, too.*

> Break down your personal barriers, and reach out
> to each other.

An old adage expresses wisdom: When you share joy it is doubled; when you share pain it is halved. Sharing your feelings will help both of you process them and feel connected.

Those Powerful Feelings

Feelings are your reaction to the world around you. They are neither positive nor negative, though they may feel this way. Your feelings are the normal and predictable responses to the cardiac crisis you have experienced and the process of recovery you are going through.

> Acknowledge and respect your feelings as real and
> important.

It's natural to put off dealing with your feelings at the height of the emergency. But the emergency is over. And your feelings probably have not disappeared. In fact, some of them may be stronger. It becomes harder to dismiss and control them as the weeks and months pass. They get in the way and intensify what may already be a difficult situation between you and your mate. Trying to manage your difficult feelings takes a great deal of energy and may strain your relationship with your mate beyond the original crisis. Ignored feelings don't go away. They often intensify and come out in unpredictable ways.

You Both Have Feelings

Though he may not have expressed it verbally, your mate is probably struggling with feelings similar to yours. Most of the professional attention he received concentrated on his physical care. Friends focus their encouragement on tangible aspects of recovery, such as improved endurance and increased strength. The scope of the patient's trauma, however, includes a threat to and a battle for his physical, emotional, mental, and spiritual life. These aspects of recovery are rarely recognized.

It is a powerful struggle for him to accept what has happened to him. Heart patients experience volatile feelings as they adapt to physical changes and limitations. Some patients manifest their anger by being demanding, withdrawn, irritable, or overly solicitous. Others demonstrate their fear by denying that anything has changed. They may continue to smoke and eat unhealthy foods. They may lift heavy objects, return to work without permission from their physicians, or push physical limits until they're exhausted. One woman insisted on vacuuming and scrubbing her kitchen floor one month after bypass surgery. She admitted to being independent and stubborn. As a result, she failed to care wisely for herself even before her incision pain had disappeared.

Most of us find it difficult to step into another person's emotional shoes. When you are in the midst of an intense experience, you cannot readily empathize with or even identify another's feelings. But trying to understand what your mate is going through is useful for three reasons: so you can see how his attitude and behavior are affecting you, so you can identify your own feelings, and so you can begin to support each other. *Because you, too, are a victim of this trauma.* Your spouse's physical heart has healed, but his battle is not yet won, nor is yours.

> State your feelings and concerns to begin a process
> of mutual recognition and validation.

Your Feelings

While it is important to take your partner's feelings into account, don't abandon your feelings for his. You best promote his recovery and yours by recognizing and respecting your own feelings.

Feelings can be divided into two general categories: "positive" and "negative," experienced as pleasurable and painful. When you experience a crisis, you suffer an emotional wound. It's common for people to try to avoid or ignore the resulting painful feelings. When something happens that is beyond personal control, people move unconsciously to what is familiar. The most common reaction to cope with an unexpected crisis is to fall back on habitual patterns of behavior.

Most of us like to think of ourselves as kind, open, and loving. We find it difficult to accept our capacity for anger and disappointment. Guilt, fear, and sadness may feel more acceptable than anger, but they, too, can be overwhelming. If you're like most heartmates, you may have thought, or even voiced, something like: "I'm trying to stay positive, but I can't stop crying" (sadness). "Why do I feel depressed when he is recovering so well?" (guilt). "I'm snapping at everyone all the time" (frustration). "It's impossible to keep my hopes up when I'm so worried" (fear). "I'm afraid I'm coming apart, and I don't know what to do about it" (anxiety/loss of control).

> Give yourself permission to *feel all* of your feelings, including the "negative" ones.

These feelings are normal. Fear, anger, sadness, and guilt are appropriate responses to the intense losses and changes you have experienced. Once you have experienced these feelings, you can begin to work with them. The first step is to recognize what they are.

Fear: The Anxiety Factory

Heartmates experience profound fears. What are they, and why are they so powerful? Abruptly and unexpectedly you find yourself in a situation that threatens all aspects of your life. Once the initial terror passes, and your partner has survived, you are faced with the unknown. Before the cardiac crisis you probably felt relatively secure and sure of yourself. Now it is nearly certain that you feel fearful—anxious and uncertain about yourself and your future.

Anxiety is defined as an intense apprehension, a fear of being hurt or losing something. All cardiac spouses are afraid of losing their partners.

This kind of fear may disrupt your normal physical or emotional functioning. It may manifest in ruminating on foreboding questions that have no answers.

Most people experience anxiety as a combination of physical symptoms mixed with an overwhelming sense of helplessness. In cases of severe anxiety, you may feel agitated, unsettled, or frantic. Your heartbeat may speed up and butterflies may flutter in your stomach. You may shake or tremble uncontrollably, sweat, get cold feet and hands. You may suffer tension headaches, react irritably, and sleep poorly. Less intense reactions include tense muscles, tightening of neck and shoulders, clenched teeth, and a vague sense of impending loss. Anxiety can be acute (short-lived and episodic) or chronic (ongoing, with varying severity).

The Fear of Being Abandoned

During the interminable hours you waited outside the hospital emergency room, wondering whether your mate was still alive, close to death, resting comfortably, or in excruciating pain, you undoubtedly asked yourself: Will my mate survive? Perhaps your anxiety was most acute at the beginning of the crisis, when everything was touch and go. Or perhaps your numbness protected you then, and now you are haunted by questions of survival. In either case, the terrible fear of being abandoned doesn't evaporate the minute your mate is discharged from the hospital. Surgical success and cardiac rehabilitation aside, no heart patient is given a clean bill of health. Consequently, all heartmates live with the anticipation and fear of a fatal episode.

I remember the terror. It began about the time my husband was due to leave the hospital. I was terrified that he would die at any moment now that we were away from the doctor and the nursing staff; terrified that he'd never recover enough to resume his place in the family as husband, father, and breadwinner; terrified that I wouldn't have the inner strength to care for him, to maintain my responsibilities as the new leader of the family. I was terrified that I felt so alone and no one seemed to know, and terrified that once he

was home everyone would abandon us, believing we no longer needed their
support or help. And, most of all, I was terrified that just thinking this way
proved that I was crazy, abnormal—had cracked under the pressure.

Your anxiety can be provoked quickly and easily. Think about how
you feel when your mate cuts your regular walk short without telling
you why. Consider your reaction when you see him "popping nitros,"
checking his pulse, taking his blood pressure. Sometimes a little
cough is all it takes to spark your anxiety.

The fear of losing your mate escalates if he doesn't seem committed to recovery. His seemingly cavalier attitude can easily frustrate
you. You become anxious about his judgment, distrusting his assessment of how much he can do. Anxiety mounts as you see that he
hasn't stopped smoking or that he is gaining weight. How can you
help but panic when he insists on shoveling snow, moving furniture,
lifting heavy boxes, or jogging too far?

It isn't unusual for heart patients to test their limits—to prove something to themselves or to want to feel useful and needed—at various
points in their recovery. Men may feel added pressure to reassert their
masculinity; women may become critical and controlling about the
way the household is being managed. It's perfectly normal for heartmates to experience periods of increased anxiety during these times.

Spiraling Anxiety

Fears about being left to cope alone spiral, producing anxiety about
your abilities in all aspects of your life. A young heartmate may not
know that she's terrified of being left alone, for example, but she experiences anxiety about her adequacy to earn a living and raise the children alone. Heartmates in their middle or later years can experience
debilitating anxiety about living alone.

Merriam, a seventy-year-old cardiac spouse, lost her first husband
to heart disease. She raised their two children alone. Once they were
grown, she began to see an old high-school sweetheart, a widower.
They married in their middle sixties, largely for companionship and

security. Merriam's second husband recently suffered a heart attack, and now she is paralyzed by her fear of being on her own. She finds it almost impossible to express her anxiety about aging and dying alone.

Since men experience heart disease earlier in life than most women, the majority of heartmates are female. Many of these women experience financial anxiety. Older women are particularly vulnerable to financial survival fears, because a large percentage have worked exclusively as homemakers or have limited their careers. Becoming a "bag lady" is a very real specter for women of any age who have not handled finances independent of their partners or not had the experience of a career. Some women describe recurring nightmares about the mortgage company appearing and threatening foreclosure. Financial anxiety can be especially poignant during times of crisis or shifts in the progress of the heart patient's recovery.

Although I have worked for most of my adult years, I felt terrified about finances after my husband's heart attack. My thinking, repetitious and negative, went something like this: "There's no way we can keep the house, we'll have to sell it. The kids have been so happy here. They'll hate living in a small apartment. There's probably not an apartment in this neighborhood that we can afford. The kids will have to change schools. How will I ever put them through college on my income alone?"

One morning, my anxiety escalated out of control. I called the social security office to ask how much money each of our children would get if their father died or was permanently disabled. Never mind that his heart attack had been described as "minor" by the doctor or that his recovery had been uncomplicated.

I was distraught. I needed information to calm me down, but then I struggled with another fear: Had I put a hex on his recovery? By thinking about money, disability, and death, I might have caused the very outcome I dreaded most, creating a sort of self-fulfilling prophecy!

Many heartmates experience acute anxiety that diminishes as their partners recover. But chronic anxiety is common for those heartmates whose partners have severe and increasingly debilitating heart disease.

Stopping the Anxiety Spiral: What You Can Do

You can take steps to cope with and alleviate your anxiety. In general, eating regular, healthy meals and getting enough sleep will help you minimize and deal with anxiety. When we don't eat right or get enough sleep, we are prone to physical and emotional stress and anxiety. The healthy changes in your partner's diet can benefit you as well. If you're having trouble sleeping, consider practicing deep-breathing exercises or other relaxation techniques (see the relaxation exercise in appendix A).

You can also tackle your anxiety emotionally and intellectually. In order to do so, you must first acknowledge that you are afraid. Fear is an emotional alarm that alerts us to defend and protect ourselves in a threatening situation. We can feel fear and anxiety about threats real or anticipated. If you ignore your anxiety and pretend that everything is fine, you short-circuit your natural warning system. You can't process your anxiety and choose to act on it or dismiss it if you don't allow yourself to recognize and accept it.

Seek the factual information you need when you are calm and when you are not experiencing anxiety. Clear, detailed information about anxiety, heart disease, recovery, finances, and other subjects related to your situation is invaluable. Your growing knowledge will help you establish a sense of understanding and safety, reduce your potential for anxiety, and aid, or enhance, your ability to cope with anxiety. Information provides a rational basis to address and process your fears.

> Address your anxiety immediately. Deal directly with the threat.

Ask yourself, "What am I afraid of? What am I afraid will happen? What am I afraid I'm losing?" Answer as rationally and as specifically as possible with the factual and experiential information you have. Seek information from others if needed. Your answers will help you perceive your situation in a new light. Then choose to accept what you cannot change, and plan ways to act on what you can change.

It is equally important to take stock of your strengths, those qualities in yourself that you can count on during an emergency or a difficult time. Look specifically at the cardiac crisis you have been through. Focus on acknowledging what you have done well. View your strengths as a resource in your plan to change what can be changed; those inner qualities will help you overcome your fears and work through your anxiety.

When Edith first came to me, she needed help managing her overwhelming fears. Her husband, Richard, had suffered several heart attacks, bypass surgery, and almost every possible complication. Edith explained that she had called 911 numerous times over the last six years. She actively worried every time she left the house, dreading another emergency, convinced that she wouldn't be there to save him. Her stomach and head ached, her muscles were tight, her speech was clipped, and her movements were agitated and jumpy. She felt frantic each time she watched Richard take his pulse or heard his audible sigh.

Edith was critical of herself because she couldn't control—or get rid of—her fear. She equated courage with fearlessness. When we talked about how strong she had been during the six years she cared for Richard, she admitted that fear had never stopped her from acting quickly or resolutely. Once Edith was able to appreciate her courage, she became more accepting of her fears.

When she hears Richard cough or sigh, Edith still experiences fear. But now, before her fears race ahead to a catastrophic conclusion, she takes a deep breath and says to herself, "I feel afraid, and I am courageous." This helps her keep her fear from overwhelming her and reminds her of her strength.

Working through Anxiety

People who have survived trauma—and cardiac spouses can be counted among them—are affected deeply. When you experience an unexpected and life-threatening event, your body instinctively goes into survival mode. Some call this reaction the fight-or-flight response. This gift of nature protects you during crises. But every gift has its benefit and its cost.

You will automatically repeat your habitual fear response every time you sense danger or a potential for loss. Your body can't differentiate between a real life-threatening crisis and a less serious event. For example, you may feel paralyzed with fear when you hear an ambulance's siren several blocks away in broad daylight. Your anxiety can be as strong as it was when you sped through the night behind the screaming ambulance that raced your mate to the hospital.

| You can learn to work through your anxiety.

You can learn to work through your automatic response, too, allowing you time to act rather than react. When you experience anxiety, concentrate first on regaining control over your body. Focus on deep breathing. It is a simple and effective way to redirect your thinking, and your increased oxygen intake will calm you naturally. If your anxiety is related to a specific concern, review the related information you have gathered. Share your thoughts and feelings with another person. These actions will reduce your catastrophic fantasies and increase your sense of control. It may be helpful to write down these steps (simplified below) and carry them in your purse or wallet.

1. Calm yourself down by taking deep breaths.
2. Engage in positive, factual self-talk (the goal is to feel safe and act functionally).
3. Reread information that you have gathered.
4. Share your thoughts and feelings with another person (there is no way to check reality in isolation).

In most cases, these techniques can help you to minimize and control your anxiety. Ask a friend or relative to listen to your fears on a regular basis. Let your confidante know that you don't expect her to fix things, that what you need is an ear, and maybe a shoulder. Sometimes anxiety can be so severe or so prolonged that professional help, including antianxiety medication, is needed. Don't hesitate to consult your own physician if you find yourself unable to handle your anxiety.

Many people find that prayers, affirmations, or poetry help them manage their anxiety. Reinhold Neibuhr's Serenity Prayer is widely used in crisis situations by people practicing Twelve-Step programs. If it fits for you, repeat it to yourself whenever you feel the need. It can be a powerful antidote to your fear and anxiety.

> *God,*
> *grant me the serenity*
> *to accept the things I cannot change,*
> *the courage to change the things I can,*
> *and the wisdom to know the difference.*

Anger: The Ogre

Are you irritated, impatient, or resentful more frequently now than before the cardiac crisis? Do you find yourself yelling at no one in particular? Are you aggravated easily for no obvious reason? If so, you are experiencing feelings of anger, as do most cardiac spouses.

Anger is a natural response during a cardiac crisis, recovery, and healing. In general, we feel anger when we perceive that an injustice has occurred, when we feel helpless about people or situations that we cannot control. These may include a wrong done to us or to others, as well as the cosmic unfairness of loss or of anticipated or unanticipated change. Our anger urges us to act and gives us the courage to do so. For people who fear the vulnerability of deep sadness, anger may be the unconscious "feeling of choice."

Why Do I Feel So Angry?

There are probably a variety of underlying triggers for your anger. It is not unusual to feel angry about situations or experiences that are beyond your control or for which there are no satisfactory explanations. You may feel anger, for example, if your partner, who diligently practices a healthy lifestyle, develops heart disease because of a genetic predisposition.

You may feel angry at the professional team that cared for your spouse at the hospital or be dissatisfied with the quality of services your spouse received. One spouse, a cardiac nurse by profession, was furious that certain drugs weren't administered to her husband. A receptionist who has put you on hold, a doctor in a hurry, or a distracted nurse who forgets to say hello are likely targets, even scapegoats, for your anger.

Some heartmates resent their partners for developing heart disease or having heart attacks. The illness or cardiac event disrupts their lives, bringing unchosen, unwanted, unpleasant, and unanticipated changes.

Josie, a cardiac spouse, described a family holiday scene. She, her husband, and their three young sons spent Thanksgiving with relatives. Even though Jack was scheduled to undergo bypass surgery the following Monday, Josie was determined to make the holiday as pleasant as possible.

All afternoon members of the family crowded around Jack, asking how he was doing and giving him their best wishes. He was the star attraction, and most of the conversation centered around his illness and impending surgery. As the day wore on, Josie became first irritated and then infuriated. She had desperately wanted Thanksgiving to be normal, especially for the sake of their children. She felt as if her life would never again be free from the focus on heart disease.

You may feel angry because your need for support is sorely neglected. Everyone expresses concern for the patient. Rarely does anyone remember to ask about you. You certainly don't begrudge him much-needed support, but it also would be nice if someone recognized your needs occasionally.

One man reported feeling like a newscaster responsible for giving up-to-the-minute reports on his wife's condition. One evening, after several such phone reports, he remembered thinking that if one more person called and asked, "How's Kathryn doing?" he would slam the phone down. He just needed someone to say, "How are you doing, Ken? I bet this is a really difficult time for you." Ken felt so outraged that he was tempted to disconnect the phone. What he really needed was a warm, human connection for himself.

If you are accustomed to relying on your spouse to meet many of your emotional needs, your feelings of neglect may well be exacerbated. You're not getting the affection or support you need right now.

You deeply miss your partner's interest in you, your daily activities, and your thoughts and ideas.

Even if he was outgoing and openly affectionate before, he may now be engrossed with his health. It seems that every time you look, he's weighing himself or taking his blood pressure. Despite your best efforts to sympathize and understand, you feel resentful at his apparent loss of interest in you and his lack of appreciation for your support and care.

Anger may be experienced and expressed without any awareness that it masks another feeling, one too difficult to be recognized. Often during cardiac recovery, anger covers deep fears or emotional pain.

Marie, a farmer's wife, reported her uncontrollable anger at Lars, her recovering spouse. She explained that her cooking style, heavy on meat and potatoes, was an accepted way to support the heavy farm work Lars did in the fields and barn . . . until he had a heart attack. Marie learned a healthier style of cooking at the hospital. She planned meals and cooked the new way with the same gusto, concern, and love as she had before.

After supper one hot summer night, Lars drove off in his pickup truck. He soon returned . . . with chocolate ice cream, which he ate ravenously, directly from the carton. Marie could not contain her anger, shouting rageful things she didn't even know she thought: how hard she had worked to save his life by changing his diet, how unappreciative he was about her efforts, and how she would leave him if he planned to slowly commit suicide by eating ice cream.

The next morning Marie could hardly believe those strong words had been hers. She was only aware of her fear that she would lose Lars.

I Shouldn't Feel Like This

Many heartmates believe that it is dangerous to the patient and their relationship to express their anger directly to the patient. They unconsciously deny their anger out of loyalty, confusion, fear, guilt, or even shame. Then, unexpectedly, uncontrolled explosions of anger may be expressed at the doctor, nursing staff, fate, or the God of their understanding. Or they may turn the anger inward (a source of depression) and berate themselves for not succeeding in making their partner live a healthier lifestyle.

Trying to explain or justify your anger is fruitless, because feelings aren't rational. Rationalizing them is like asking yourself if it is all right to be hungry or thirsty. Like hunger and thirst, feelings exist and are normal responses to your situation. You don't need to justify your feelings to yourself or to anyone else (feelings are only feelings). Your anger is a signal that you are experiencing a crisis. Anger, according to Stephanie Ericsson, can help you express your needs.

> [Anger is] natural protective armor. It tells the rest of the world that a boundary has been violated. Our society would have us swallow it, and many of us do. . . . Rage is white-hot anger. . . . It is a superb emotion. Used correctly, it lays down permanent boundaries, stakes out lifetime territories, and gives us girth. It will launch us out of inertia and thrust us forward.[2]

Getting angry is *not* dangerous to your spouse's health. Of course, I'm not suggesting that you berate your mate during the first forty-eight hours after a heart attack. Nor do I advocate that you take advantage of the situation to rage or act like a nasty ogre or a spoiled brat. Both you and your mate are experiencing angry feelings about all the changes that heart disease has created in your lives. Your anger doesn't mean that you don't love each other. You can find appropriate ways to express your anger and learn how to diffuse it.

Expressing Your Anger
Direct communication is usually the safest and most effective way to express anger to your mate. But it is important to allow yourself time to first feel your anger and then think about it before you communicate it. This can help you clarify how you feel, which may reduce some of the intensity of the anger. Then you can determine what you choose to say, if anything.

There are many different ways you can manage your anger. Some people release it physically. You can pound the wall, swim laps vigorously, or smash a tennis ball or racquetball. Yell into a pillow or shout in the shower—just raising your voice is a great release. Some people release their anger by writing about it. Others find it helpful to share their feelings with a trusted friend.

You may still feel the need to air your anger directly with your partner. But deciding to do so can feel threatening, especially if it is unprecedented in your relationship. Here are some suggestions for negotiating such a discussion. They provide safety for both of you and a foundation on which to build further communication.

- Make a pact that allows for the honest expression of anger.
- Choose a place for discussion that is comfortable and private.
- Commit to listening fully and openly.
- Set a time limit (five minutes may be sufficient) for each of you to speak.
- Agree not to interrupt; take turns speaking.
- Remember that you are on the same team and that you love each other.

The following "dos" and "don'ts" checklist can also help you express your anger safely and effectively.

HEARTMATES® ANGER CHECKLIST

Do	Don't
Do say what hurts	Don't avoid talking about important issues
Do begin all angry statements with "I"	Don't use your anger to blame
Do use your anger to clear the air	Don't mistake anger for violence or aggression
Do try to make yourself understood	Don't exaggerate, whine, or complain
Do tell it straight	Don't rationalize or intellectualize
Do say what you think	Don't save up little irritations until your anger explodes
Do say regularly how you feel	Don't withdraw for fear you'll injure your mate
Do raise your voice until you're heard	Don't believe your relationship is too fragile to bear the weight of your feelings
Do take responsibility; "own" your anger	Don't sacrifice your anger in exchange for physical symptoms like headaches, TMJ, or depression
Do say you're angry	Don't use your anger to attack or punish your mate

Sadness: The Heavy Weight

It may seem strange to feel sad at a time like this. Your mate is recovering. You should be happy, right? And you probably are. But major life changes, even good changes, normally include sadness, heartache, and even depression.

We all tend to take our lives for granted. When something happens that jeopardizes our security, we experience enormous feelings of loss. We grieve. In a cardiac crisis, all that you hold near and dear has been threatened. The everyday freedom and long-term security you counted on suddenly seems tenuous, or even lost. It is normal to feel sad, even depressed, about these changes and losses.

Recognizing Sadness and Depression

You may recognize sadness by its effects on your body. The physical counterparts sometimes appear as lethargy or fatigue. Cardiac spouses often attempt to hide their sadness for fear of appearing ungrateful, selfish, insensitive, or weak. In the hospital and during the early recovery period, you may have "put on a happy face" and worn a mask of cheerfulness and confidence that you didn't feel. As you relax your pose, you may feel sad. Your sadness may range in intensity from cheerlessness and downheartedness to sorrow and melancholy.

Janet, age thirty-nine, described her life before her husband's heart attack. She jokingly referred to herself as the "tour director." She constantly organized social activities for the two of them and their friends. They were enthusiastic sports fans and patrons of the local art museum and repertory theater. They made several business trips and took vacations each year. Making arrangements was almost a full-time job for Janet.

Since Brendan's bypass surgery, Janet wanders through her immaculate condominium pondering the purpose of her life. The structure of her daily routine has toppled. Accustomed to organizing and taking charge, Janet feels lost, aimless, and adrift. She is wary of feeling sorry for herself because she has always felt so privileged. But her old life is gone. Her new life is still a question mark. The void leaves her feeling empty, confused, and sad.

Few cardiac spouses have lost such an exciting and romantic way of life, but all confront the disappointment of broken dreams. Margaret, a careful and conservative person, and her husband, Patrick, planned to realize a lifelong dream and retire to a quiet, rural town somewhere in a warm climate. Just one year before retiring from his construction job, Patrick suffered a severe heart attack. Their savings have dwindled because of medical and related expenses. Margaret empathizes with Patrick's fear and understands his need to stay in Wisconsin, where his doctor and family members can give him the support he needs. Still, she mourns the loss of her retirement cottage in the sun.

Heartmates experience many frustrated expectations. If your mate has a second heart attack or a setback during recovery, for example, both of you may feel lower than you did at the onset of the first cardiac event. Your mate's physical recovery may be more complicated and prolonged the second time around. Your sadness may be, too. It takes more effort to feel optimistic and to trust the medications, recovery program, and even your doctor when you have to start all over again.

Pamela's outlook, for example, was very positive when Jerry returned to work after recovering from his first heart attack. But she described her attitude after his second heart attack and surgery as negative, even despairing. She had a very hard time accepting his forced retirement when he was only fifty-eight.

Some of the sadness that cardiac spouses report indicates yearning for things past: Christmas as it used to be when he dressed up like Santa to pass out gifts to the children or grandchildren; those few years comparatively free of responsibility after the children were grown and before his heart attack; long driving trips across the country every summer until his cardiac surgery. Since the onset of heart disease, each holiday, every season, is an occasion for gratitude and grieving.

Sometimes normal sadness deepens into depression. Symptoms of depression can creep up slowly, or hit you early and hard. Depression saps your energy and reduces your ability to function. You may feel as if nothing matters or that it takes all of your stamina just to get through the day. You may even question the meaning and purpose of your life.

Working through Sadness and Depression

I remember the audible sigh of relief in the room when a cardiologist, speaking to a group of patients and spouses, acknowledged that it is normal for cardiac patients to experience depression.[3] The same is true for heartmates and other cardiac family members. And your sadness or depression is manageable.

To deal with your sadness or depression, you must acknowledge it and mourn your loss or losses to completion. Let yourself grieve. Doing so may seem difficult and painful, even frightening. But disregarding your feelings won't make them go away.

> Grieve your losses to completion. Only then can you move to acceptance, peace, and healing.

You may find social pressure makes it difficult to experience your feelings fully. Our society supports quick decisions and avoidance of pain.[4] But each person is unique, experiencing grief differently and at an individual pace. Resist outside pressure and the temptation to avoid your pain. Don't feel that you have to be finished with your sadness or disappointment according to someone else's schedule. Don't be pressured by comments about "dwelling on your sadness" or implications that you should "hurry up and get on with your life."

One Sunday afternoon about two months after my husband's heart attack, a friend invited me to join her at the movies. It sounded like the perfect thing to do to get away. But when it was time to get ready, I felt exhausted and wondered why I'd agreed to the outing.

I was surprised and disturbed when I couldn't keep my mind on the film. Everyone in the theater laughed out loud, but I didn't find the clever dialogue at all funny. I couldn't concentrate on or analyze any of the ideas.

It was just too early for me to enjoy myself. I couldn't escape my sadness. In the grand scheme of things, the movie seemed trivial in comparison with my personal struggles. I returned home feeling sad and alienated from life.

It's a myth that "acting happy" will speed your partner through his sadness or depression or his physical recovery. It certainly won't help you. Feeling sad is a very natural part of your humanity. By feeling and experiencing your grief, you promote healing and make yourself more available for your mate's recovery. As the Gospel tells us, "Blessed are those who mourn, for they shall be comforted" (Matthew 5:4).

In time, your sadness will diminish. You'll know naturally when you've grieved enough. Your physical, emotional, and mental energy will return. You may suddenly feel motivated to do things that for months have seemed impossible. You will find yourself spontaneously interested in others again. Your focus will shift from yearning for a lost past to the present moment and to planning for your future with renewed enthusiasm.

If your sadness doesn't lift and you continue to have difficulty functioning after the early months of recovery, you are likely experiencing depression. Seek professional counsel or a referral from your doctor.

Guilt: The Iron Grip

Guilt is a complicated feeling often motivated by another feeling. If you feel angry at your mate who's been sick or nearly died, or you feel sad about the loss of your own dream since his heart disease, you may then feel guilty about having those feelings. But feelings aren't rational. Your anger, sadness, and guilt are real and normal.

Sometimes guilt covers up feelings that are less acceptable to you. You may feel guilty because you think your feelings are selfish, wrong, or different from what is expected. At other times, you feel guilty when you realize you've done something hurtful to another person and you feel disappointed in yourself.

Am I Guilty?

Many cardiac spouses feel responsible for their mate's heart disease. Louise, an assertive and outspoken woman, suffered guilt for many months because she and Jay had been arguing when his chest pain began. As she waited and watched in the hospital, she became convinced that if she hadn't raised her voice, hadn't felt so righteous about expressing her opinion, her darling Jay would not be in cardiac care. Even the lectures she attended at the hospital that helped define risk factors and methods of prevention did nothing to free Louise from her belief that she had caused Jay's heart attack. She couldn't look at the scar on Jay's chest, because it was such a powerful reminder of her fault.

Louise's case may seem extreme, but consider all the ways you feel responsible. You may feel guilty for using so much salt in your cooking over the last thirty years. One man felt guilty because he agreed to his wife's demand to drive her to the hospital rather than call 911. He believed that the damage to his wife's heart was increased because he lost precious minutes en route. Many spouses feel guilty because they didn't try to intervene in their mate's hospital care. Others feel especially guilty because they enjoy good health while their mate has heart disease. They may even try to hide how well they feel so their spouse won't feel envious.[5]

Still others suffer because they were unsuccessful at initiating intervention. This was dramatized in the television movie *Heartsounds* (adapted from Martha Weinman Lear's book of the same title), when a cardiac spouse confronted the night nurse to persuade her to wake the intern to change orders. The nurse refused because she was afraid she'd lose her job.

You probably know that in reality you did the best you could in trying circumstances. You realize that blaming yourself is unreasonable, but understanding that doesn't make your guilt automatically disappear. Holding on to unrealistic guilt about what you did or didn't do can become a slippery slope leading to shame, a state in which you believe that you, not just your feelings or actions, are bad. But you can discern and use your guilt for good in your recovery and in relation to your partner as well.

Managing Your Guilt
What can you do about your guilt? First you can examine it to determine whether it is real and realistic. If it isn't, you will find that it is

masking a deeper feeling. Then you can focus your attention on the primary feeling. If your guilt is real, it functions like a wake-up call. Real guilt often points out that you are acting contrary to your values. It can signal that you have or are treating someone poorly, unfairly, unjustly. Once you are aware of it, you can make appropriate amends.

In either case, guilt can be experienced as a positive opportunity because it gives you valuable information about your feelings and actions. With such awareness, you are in a position to decide how you can respond more authentically. Once you've examined your guilt you can let it go.

Guilt becomes a problem when it's misunderstood. Well-wishers all around you are cheering for your mate's recovery. What kind of a person would risk sabotaging the patient's progress by expressing worry or fear? What sort of individual feels sad and depressed when everyone else is acting cheerful and optimistic?

> When you feel guilty about your feelings, examine them. Find out where your worry and disappointment are coming from. Examine your sadness or anger. Understand how you have been hurt and experience those feelings fully.

Your feelings are normal and you are not a bad person for feeling the way you do. If you feel guilty about hurting your spouse, assess your realistic responsibility.[6] Be accountable for your actions; apologize and make appropriate amends if the situation permits. Remember, your spouse's physical heart has healed. Your thoughts and feelings will not damage it.

Working with Changing Feelings

It's easy to be overwhelmed by your emotions in a crisis. Even after a crisis has passed, feelings can be tricky and perplexing. It may be difficult to sort out your feelings, much less determine if they require any action. This feelings inventory will help you understand and cope with your feelings. It will also be a valuable tool for managing your feelings, helping you act rather than react to them.

HEARTMATES® FEELINGS INVENTORY

Step 1: Stop and take time to recognize what you are feeling. Labeling your feelings, one by one, you can begin to clarify them.

Step 2: Figure out what it is, if anything, that your feelings are telling you about what you need to take care of yourself. What, for example, would help to reduce or resolve your feelings of fear, sadness, anger, and guilt? What are your feelings telling you that you need?

Step 3: Once you have determined what you need, you can take action to get your need met in appropriate ways. Creative solutions may require using your imagination and holding a positive attitude.

One way to keep yourself on track with this exercise is to put it in writing. Consider using the Heartmates Feelings and Needs Assessment Diary regularly for several weeks.[7]

As your feelings and needs change over time, you may find a weekly, and then monthly, evaluation helpful. The pages of your diary may follow the form I suggest here:

HEARTMATES®
FEELINGS AND NEEDS ASSESSMENT DIARY

Feelings	Needs	Solutions

1. Under Feelings, write down a feeling you are experiencing that concerns you. (Begin the sentence with "I feel. . . .")
2. Under Needs, write down a need you have that is related to that feeling. (Begin the sentence with "I need. . . .")
3. Under Solutions, write down as many actions as you can think of that can satisfy your need. (Begin each sentence with "I could. . . .")

Here are some sample entries:

- I feel scared about money. I need information about our health benefits. . . . I could call our accountant. I could call the social security office. I could look at our budget and financial records from last year. I could ask my partner to discuss our financial situation with me.
- I feel irritable about everything. I need some time for myself. . . . I could take a nap. I could stay out of the kitchen and go to a restaurant for dinner tonight. I could weed my garden. I could make a cup of tea and sit down to read my favorite magazine. I could take a warm bubble bath. I could go for a long walk in the park. I could go sit in the chapel.

- I feel afraid of being alone. I need to belong, to feel connected. . . . I could call one of our kids to arrange a visit. I could take a walk with my spouse. I could go to lunch with my best friend. I could reach out to talk to my next-door neighbor. I could arrange to do some volunteer work with others through my church or community center.
- I feel sad. I need to give myself time and attention to express my feelings. . . . I could have a good cry. I could write a sad poem. I could ask my mate to hold me. I could share my sadness with a dear friend.

The Heartmates Feelings and Needs Assessment Diary doesn't include space for the last step in the process: *choose* one of your solutions and do it. Commit yourself to making your solution a reality.

The last step often involves asking for what you want from other people. For most of us, this is difficult. But if you are willing to reach out—to your mate, to other family members, to friends—you will have a better chance of having your needs met.

Seeking Support

Working your way through a crisis or difficult life change is a highly personal experience. Think of how often you have sat up late at night worrying about your mate's health and wondering about your future. You may fear for your sanity because one minute you feel totally withdrawn from relationships and the next you desperately seek closeness. You may have thought that no one understands what you're going through. You're right. It's impossible for anyone to completely comprehend your experience. But that doesn't mean that no one cares.

There are times when solitude is exactly what you need. The soul-searching done when you are alone can be peaceful and healing. But you also need support. When you are hurting, it is especially important to allow yourself to be cared for.

Each of us finds comfort in different ways. Express your fear and frustration to someone who is willing to listen patiently without making judgments. The kind word or warm hug you receive can be a much-needed gift of support. Or you may take solace from simply being in the company of a close friend.

Your friends and family may or may not be as supportive as you like or had anticipated. Even those who try their best may fail to offer their support in ways that seem right to you. But look closer. Family, friends—even your higher power—may be at work in your life in ways you hadn't noticed.

David, a most pious man, climbed onto his roof during a flood. A boat going up the river stopped to invite him aboard. David refused, thanking them, because he believed God would provide.

He continued to sit on the roof and the water rose above the windows of his home. Another boat came by carrying people to dry land upstream, and they shouted up to him that they had room for him. Again, David declined, citing his belief that God would save him. The water rose up to the shingles of his roof.

A helicopter flew by, saw David, and offered him a ladder to climb aboard. He responded, "Take your people to safety; I am not afraid, God will provide."

By dusk, all but the peak of his roof was covered and the water was lapping at David's feet, and he cried, "God, why have you forsaken me?" There was a deafening thunderclap, and a voice from the sky declared, "I didn't forsake you, David. Who do you think sent you two boats and a helicopter?"

This parable shows that support is often available to you. To see it, you may need to follow these simple guidelines: Remember that those who sit passively waiting usually miss the boat! Stay flexible. Assess and reassess what you are getting from others. It may be exactly what you need, but not what you want. Support may not come packaged as you expect it. You need to do your part.

People in your life may unwittingly contribute to your sense of isolation despite their good intentions. Early in the crisis, friends and family are apt to check in often. Their first question is about your partner's health. And rightly so. They express relief that he's doing well and recovering quickly. Most conversations end with the statement:

"You must be thrilled that everything is going so well." Their concern is appreciated, but it's hardly an invitation to express your needs.

| Be proactive; ask for what you need.

It's not easy to ask a friend or relative for support, especially when they don't offer it directly. If your relationship is not characterized by sharing and intimacy, you may feel uncomfortable exposing your vulnerability. Realize that *this is an extraordinary situation*. Normal rules of etiquette don't apply. Your friends and family may be unsure of appropriate ways to approach you. Perhaps they, too, present a cheerful face in order to keep up your spirits—and their own.

Your need for someone to listen to you lovingly and without judgment is real—especially when you are in a crisis. You are fortunate if you know someone who supports you in that way. Most people slip from loving listening to frantic fixing as soon as your pain resonates inside them. When they realize they've failed to give you the magic answer, they hesitate to listen again. Ask others for what you need clearly and directly.

> State your needs clearly and directly. Doing so will eliminate guesswork and increase the potential for your needs being met.

There's an old "Peanuts" cartoon strip in which Marcie hears her friend, Peppermint Patty, bemoaning how poorly she was doing in school. Marcie launches into a litany of advice: "Go to bed earlier, eat a better breakfast—" but Peppermint Patty interrupts. "You've never understood, have you, Marcie, that when a person complains, he doesn't want a solution, he wants sympathy!" Sometimes all we need is a sympathetic ear, but others can't know that unless we tell them.

I remember a call from my daughter, Deb. She was calling from college, hundreds of miles away. I heard her voice, sobbing through the wires, and knew she needed my help. Talking through her tears, she told me what was wrong.

As I listened, my mind flew through my trusty list of therapeutic solutions. She paused, but only temporarily, to catch her breath, wipe her tears. I jumped into the silence with my first suggestion. She interrupted me, in a voice only a daughter uses with her mother: "I know what to do about it. I called so you would listen to me cry." What a relief and what a wonderful lesson for me. All she needed was her mother's sympathetic ear!

If you feel uneasy expressing your feelings or find it difficult to do so clearly, experiment a little, test the waters. Share one personal thing the next time a friend, relative, or neighbor calls. Once the initial barrier is broken, it will be easier to do it again.

> Make it a habit to share something personal once each day. Assess how it goes. Don't overdo it. Take small steps.

If you take the risk and ask for support, you may be pleasantly surprised by how eagerly it's given. It's also important to accept the gestures of support you receive; it's how your needs get met. Accepting offers of meals or even financial aid from relatives is a way of letting people be there for you. Asking a friend to stop over for an hour so that you can take a break is not an imposition in a time of crisis. One day you may have the opportunity to return the favor.

Reaching Out

Some of the best support you find may be with someone who is going through a similar experience. Other cardiac spouses are uniquely capable of relating to your feelings.

On the day of my husband's bypass surgery, I shared the waiting room with another cardiac spouse and her family. As the minutes crawled by, we each sat silently, alone with our thoughts. Finally, the door opened. The chaplain walked over and stood in front of me. Placing his hand on my shoulder, he said, "Your husband has come through fine; the surgery is over." My eyes filled with tears of relief. And through my tears, I saw that the other cardiac spouse was weeping, too.

During that seemingly unending block of time, we shared an intimacy that I'll never forget. The experience of the strong bond that developed so quickly between us forcefully reminded me that I was not alone. Later we kept each other company outside Intensive Care and visited each other's husbands in the postsurgical unit. Once we left the hospital, we went our separate ways. But, in a very special way, we will always be connected.

Meet other cardiac spouses by attending educational programs sponsored by your local hospital or clinic. In addition, your community may have support groups for people affected by disease or trauma. These groups offer you a place to share your story, as well as fellowship, perspective, and guidance.

At times it becomes necessary to reach out to mental health professionals. Seeking this help does not mean you are weak or that you have failed; it means that you respect and honor yourself. Professional counseling during a time of crisis can be an important means of support and healing. Choose a professional who is knowledgeable about and sensitive to your needs.

Remember, ultimately, that *you are not alone.* Reaching out for support is an absolutely essential step in your recovery and in the process of reclaiming your health—and your life.[8]

A FEW POINTS TO REMEMBER ABOUT FEELINGS

- Feelings exist. You are not responsible for how you feel.
- It is normal to experience fear, anger, sadness, and guilt in response to the cardiac crisis.
- Depression is a normal response to a cardiac event for patients, spouses, and other family members.
- Recognizing and identifying your feelings relieves and empowers you.

- Feelings provide an important source of information about yourself and your reactions to the world around you.
- Feelings change over time.
- Accepting and understanding your feelings gives you options about how and when to express them.
- Your feelings make you human and unique.
- Feelings connect you to other human beings.

Chapter 3 Notes

1. For further understanding about the loneliness of the heartmate, see the essay in appendix C in this book. For a clarifying and consoling book on the subject, read *Ambiguous Loss: Learning to Live with Unresolved Grief,* by Pauline Boss (Cambridge, Mass.: Harvard University Press, 1999).
2. See Stephanie Ericsson's *Companion through the Darkness: Inner Dialogues on Grief* (New York: HarperCollins, 1993) for an eloquent and elegant experience of grieving. Her perspective on the utility of anger can be found on page 61 of this book.
3. See a study reported in the April 25, 2000 *Circulation: Journal of the American Heart Association* about social support and depression in heart patients. Also, a 1996 *Wall Street Journal* article, "Treating Depression Gives Heart Patients Better Chance at Life," indicates that depression affects about 50 percent of the million heart attack survivors and 30 to 40 percent of the 350,000 bypass patients annually. An editorial from October 1993 in *The Journal of the American Medical Association* said it was unethical for cardiac depression to be left untreated!
4. Lesley Hazelton, *The Right to Feel Bad* (New York: Ballantine Books, 1984), 196–97.
5. The importance of the well spouse maintaining her health and her own separate life is discussed by Maggie Strong in her book *Mainstay: For the Well Spouse of the Chronically Ill* (Boston: Little, Brown, & Co., 1988).
6. It is useful to differentiate between needless guilt and healthy, appropriate guilt. See Judith Viorst, "Good as Guilt," chapter 9 in her book *Necessary Losses* (New York: Fawcett Gold Medal, 1986), 150–51, for a discussion on the healing value of making reparations for a wrongful act. Consider a Twelve-Step recovery program. Major elements of recovery are taking a

"fearless moral inventory" and "making amends." Also, read the sections on forgiveness in chapters 6 and 10 of this book.

7. The Heartmates Feelings and Needs Assessment Diary is adapted from Ellen Sue Stern's *Expecting Change* (New York: Poseidon Press, 1986), 114–15.

8. Being alone is basic to the process of grief that all heartmates encounter, but aloneness must be differentiated from loneliness. When the heartmate reaches out to tell someone her story and ask for support, she breaks through loneliness and experiences connection and belonging to the human community. Being vulnerable and sharing deep experiences with another person is a building block in establishing community. See appendix C of this book for a deeper look at loneliness and its antidotes.

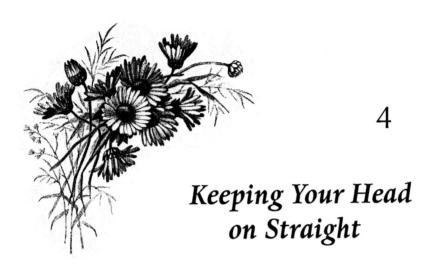

4

Keeping Your Head
on Straight

A cardiac event affects the workings of your mind every bit as much as your feelings. It can play havoc with your thinking long after the immediate crisis is past.

From the first instant, everything feels as though it's happening in double time. In a state of shock, you try desperately to clear your head and make the right moves. Inundated with information and advice, you struggle to make sense of it all. As you try to comprehend what's happened and what's happening, you may be surprised by your inability to think straight.

You may feel as if you've lost control or gone crazy. You haven't. It is common and normal for heartmates to have trouble concentrating, processing, and retaining information, as well as making judgments and decisions. You have experienced trauma and are responding as we all do when confronted with a frightening, life-threatening, and life-changing event.

In the first days after my husband's heart attack, my mind seemed to have a life of its own. I was plagued by an incessant litany of unanswerable questions. Instead of thinking, "Well, I can see I'm in an awful situation; I need to figure out what to do," I fixated on the same material, my mind like a race car careening wildly around and around a circular track.

The logical questions I wish I could have asked were: "What is the pri-ority here? What do I need to think about right now? What questions do I need to ask? What plans should I be considering? What do I need to do today, this minute?"

What You Need to Know
about Your Thinking

It usually takes time, sometimes as much as several months, for your mind to return to its normal level of functioning. Some cardiac spouses have chronic problems concentrating and remembering details, because they are still so preoccupied. One woman, who had always been a voracious reader, couldn't focus her attention long enough to follow magazine recipes for the first six months after her mate's heart attack. Another spouse had to bring work home with him. His shortened attention span caused him to fall behind on the job.

I was particularly unnerved by an incident that showed how distracted I was. One day several weeks after my husband's heart attack, I was driving home from work. When I turned off the ignition, I was surprised to find myself in the driveway of our old house. We hadn't lived there for more than two years. I must have been driving on automatic pilot, or maybe I uncon-sciously wanted to turn back the clock to a simpler time. In either case, I felt scared by how disoriented I was. I wondered if it was safe for me to drive. I even thought I might be going crazy.

Another phenomenon that is instinctively triggered when people con-front sudden and unexpected loss is called "life review."[1] The most important events of your life are instantaneously recalled. You may experience this when you avert a driving accident; your whole life flashes in front of you before you brake to a halt.

Recall getting the news of your spouse's heart attack. You may have experienced a partial life review in that moment: a review that highlighted your whole marriage. You may have lost track of time momentarily or been thoroughly absorbed in another world while this was happening. None of this means that you've lost your mind. On the contrary, life review is a natural process that prepares us to deal with change and loss.

Circular thinking is another symptom that affects cardiac spouses. Like a broken record, your mind repeats the events of this family crisis. You may go over and over the same stories, lose your train of thought, or be totally unable to think about anything else. You may find this repetitive thinking occurring for many weeks into the recovery period. Your normal thinking process should return after you recognize and examine what has happened and how it has affected you. It takes time for people to get their hearts and minds around monumental changes.

It is normal and healthy to relive your experience. Your mind is trying to make sense of shocking and chaotic events. Mental repetition can bring order out of chaos. By repeating the details of your experience aloud, you clarify and deepen your understanding and move toward acceptance.

You will probably experience an urgent need to share your experience with others over and over again. Sharing serves a purpose; it may even be the necessary foundation for integrating your experience, recovering from the cardiac crisis, and continuing your personal growth. In his classic work about coping with life changes, William Bridges emphasizes that "you cannot really terminate anything without reviewing it and putting it into order."[2] While your need to share your experience will probably diminish over time, cardiac spouses exchange stories for years and with as much intensity as if the events had just happened. Be gentle and patient with yourself. Be sure to give yourself as much time as you need to share, process, and heal.

Meeting with other heartmates is a good outlet for sharing. Sharing with them one-to-one or in a group will give you the opportunity to tell your story to a receptive and supportive audience long after friends and neighbors have lost interest.

Clearly, surviving the acute crisis doesn't automatically relieve the stresses and pressures that exist. A number of responsibilities follow you home from the hospital. You must be attentive and alert to communicate with the doctor, supervise your mate's medications, and structure a new dietary plan. Beyond coping with daily tasks, you need your mind clear to make ongoing decisions and to confront the deeper meaning of the crisis.

Untangling the Web

Your thoughts and your feelings are closely intertwined. Anxiety can strangle your thinking. When you're not thinking rationally, your anxiety accelerates and the two become a vicious cycle.

You "may experience intense emotion but without clear memory of the [cardiac] event, or may remember everything in detail but without emotion." This explains the "severing of the normal connections of memory, knowledge, and emotion resulting from intense emotional reactions to traumatic events," according to Dr. Judith Herman in her classic study of trauma.[3]

In a crisis, powerful feelings wrap themselves around your mind like a blanket, suffocating it. No matter how hard you try to concentrate, you end up panicky and confused. Fears about the future paralyze you until you can't think. Even after you make a decision, fear can stop you, freezing your action.

If you're blaming yourself for not being more organized and decisive, *stop*. It's very likely that your feelings are getting in the way. Whether you seek information, have an important decision to make, or need solutions to more unanswered questions, first deal with your feelings. Acknowledging your feelings is important. If you know what you're feeling, you may be able to calm down, begin to think clearly, and free yourself to take appropriate action.

Gathering information is a positive way to cope with your feelings and dispel anxiety. Most people cope better when they have the whole story. Without it, your imagination runs wild, creating scenarios far worse than reality. If you're like most cardiac spouses, you probably have a slew of unspoken, unaddressed, and unanswered questions. They may torment you when you are trying to sleep or pop up at odd times, catching you unaware. You may find them circling around and around in your head, leaving you feeling as if you're enmeshed in a web.

> You can take control of your concerns. To help you
> untangle your web of questions, keep a pad of
> paper and a pen or pencil handy, day and night.
> Write down any question that comes into your
> mind.

You also can ask your questions aloud to yourself or to someone willing to listen.

Organizing Your Questions

Once you have access to your questions, separate them into two groups: those that are unanswerable and those that have potential answers. Set aside the questions that don't have answers. In order to reduce your anxiety and empower yourself toward action, focus on questions that can be answered. (Using your mind will reassure you that you haven't lost it.) You can then further organize your answerable questions by dividing them into two subgroups: informational questions and decision-making questions.

Informational questions provide data about your mate's condition, prognosis, and the ongoing realities of living with someone who has a chronic, life-threatening illness. This information can help you assess your situation. Some sample informational questions include:

- What causes heart disease?
- What are the newest medical treatments that may prolong my partner's life?
- How long will recovery take?
- What lifestyle limitations can we anticipate?
- When is it safe to resume sexual activity?

Obtaining information is an ongoing process. Attend lectures and participate in seminars for cardiac patients and their families. Not only may you get answers to your questions, but you might learn something that will directly improve your spouse's recovery. Cardiac rehabilitation programs at your local hospital, YMCA, or Jewish Community Center can be a rich resource for practical, up-to-date information.

If you aren't accustomed to being persistent and assertive, you may find that seeking information is difficult but empowering. If you have been hesitant to ask others, especially other heartmates or qualified professionals, about highly personal things, try not to let fear or embarrassment stop you from finding out what you need to know. Summoning your courage to discuss sexual activity with your physician, for example, may be important to guide your return to physical intimacy. (See chapter 8, "Re-pairing the Heartmate Connection," for information on sexuality and other aspects of repairing your disrupted relationship.) Steadying your mind and seeking answers to your questions will increase your confidence in yourself as you journey through recovery.

You also can conduct research on your own (though it can be beneficial to verify your findings with others). Trips to the library for the most current data and new developments in cardiac care will yield valuable information. Make sure, however, that you consult current books and journals. Much has changed, and continues to change, in the diagnosis and treatment of heart disease.

> Research reliable health sites on the Web for current information on heart disease, treatments, maintenance, and spiritual and psychological concerns, as well as offer connection to other heartmates.

Please note that there is a great deal of outdated, misleading, unsubstantiated, and incorrect information on the Web. Stick with reliable sources and try to find more than one source to substantiate your findings. Start your research using your favorite search engines. The Heartmates Web site is another good starting place, offering a wealth of updated information <www.heartmates.com>.

STARTING POINTS

Contact or visit any of the following organizations. What you learn may benefit you and your mate directly. Seeking, getting, and understanding information on heart disease and recovery can help you focus your thinking, strengthen your foundation for decision making, reduce your feelings of helplessness, and increase your sense of safety and control.

American Association of Cardiovascular
  and Pulmonary Rehabilitation (AACVPR)
401 Michigan Avenue, Suite 2200
Chicago, Illinois 60611
(312) 321-5146
www.aacvpr.org

American Heart Association (National Center)
7320 Greenville Avenue
Dallas, Texas 75231
(800) 242-8721
(888) 694-3278
www.americanheart.org
(Use your phone book to locate your state office.)

Harvard Heart Letter
(a monthly newsletter from Harvard Medical School)
10 Shattuck Street
Boston, Massachusetts 02115
www.health.harvard.edu

Heartmates
P.O. Box 16202
Minneapolis, Minnesota 55416
(952) 929-3331; fax (952) 929-6395
heartmates@heartmates.com
www.heartmates.com

National Family Caregivers Association
(a national network of well spouses of the chronically ill)
10400 Connecticut Avenue, Suite 500
Kensington, Maryland 20895
www.nfcacares.org

WomenHeart, the National Coalition for
  Women with Heart Disease
818 18th Street NW, Suite 730
Washington, DC 20006
(202) 728-7199
www.womenheart.org

Decision-making questions have a different purpose from informational questions. They are geared to help you think about issues so you can make informed decisions. Some sample decision-making questions include:

- How should I tell family members about a change in my spouse's condition?
- Should my spouse go ahead with bypass surgery?
- What financial adaptations do we need to make?
- What changes need I consider about my career or retirement?
- What lifestyle changes should we make? Should I make?
- Should we still make vacation plans for the coming year?

Gathering and Organizing Information

The wealth of information available to you and the task of gathering and organizing it can be overwhelming. Share the responsibility. Delegate some of the research tasks to family members. They will feel included, an important part of the family team, and will reduce your sense of impossible burden in this crisis. Further, cooperation aids the development of family skills. When difficult issues arise, family members have a head start on feeling included, are better able to communicate, and can better participate in making decisions that will affect the whole family.

Gather information to be used "in case of emergency." Make a list of sources, people who need to be notified or consulted in an emergency. Include people who are likely to be helpful and available, noting the type of assistance they are able to provide. Collect phone and pager numbers, as well as street and e-mail addresses of medical resources, social service agencies, and financial resource institutions in your city.

Maintain a current and organized bank of important information. Keep an updated medical history and medications profile. Generate a list of medical emergency contacts, too. Organize important family documents. Include wills, living wills (or signed durable powers of attorney), advance directives, and spiritual-ethical wills.[4]

Inform family members where this information can be found. You might consider making copies of the information bank to give to family members. You could, for example, use notebooks or ring binders that can be updated. Keep the master copy in a prominent place in your home.

If we could know the unknown, if there were perfect solutions, we wouldn't ever experience crises. The best we can do is prepare as thoroughly as we can. Involve all your family members, including the patient, and know that this information-gathering process will give you and your family a clearer sense of priorities, safety, and control, as well as a share in hope and love.

Accentuate the Positive

Heartmates often feel depressed and pessimistic even after the doctor indicates that a high quality of life is the most likely prognosis for the patient. You don't have to stay stuck with your negative reactions. You can learn skills to clarify your thinking, enhance your recovery experience, and renew your sense of safety. Martin E. P. Seligman, who has studied helplessness and pessimism juxtaposed with empowerment and optimism, explains:

When we encounter adversity, we react by thinking about it. Our thoughts rapidly congeal into beliefs. . . . Usually the negative beliefs that follow adversity are inaccurate. . . . These beliefs may become so habitual we don't even realize we have them unless we stop and focus on them. And they don't just sit there idly; they have consequences. The beliefs are the direct causes of what we feel and what we do next.[5]

The key to changing your thinking pattern requires you to analyze *how* you think. You may not be experienced at such analysis, but you can learn. Here are four steps designed to assist you. Follow them to gain control and the ability to use your thinking to positively affect your future.

1. Gather and evaluate all the evidence supporting your beliefs. Verify the accuracy of what you tell yourself. This technique involves asking yourself the question: What is the evidence for my belief? Factual evidence that points out the distortions in your catastrophic thoughts and beliefs is essential to transforming them. Look for the evidence that shifts your focus away from unfounded, ungrounded, reactionary suppositions to grounded, balanced, thinking.

You might, for example, believe that your healthy food plan is shot and that another cardiac event is imminent. Why? Because your spouse ate chocolate cake and ice cream at a family birthday party. Look at all the evidence. Count the actual fat grams and calories your mate consumed at the party. Reread results of his latest cholesterol tests, and acknowledge weight loss by noting what the bathroom scale reads. Put the alleged crime in perspective.

2. When something automatically triggers your pessimistic beliefs, look at a variety of potential causes for the event. This will help you get beyond your initial assumptions so you can stop focusing on only the most catastrophic possibilities. Scan your understanding for the possible reasons for the event, looking for those that are changeable, specific, and nonpersonal. Your task is to identify alternative causes,

rather than succumb to the old habit of latching onto the most negative ones.

During that cake-eating incident, for example, remind yourself that maintaining total deprivation of favorite foods is impossible for long periods of time. This understanding can ease your "dis-ease" when your mate eats cake and ice cream during a family birthday party. Taking a break from your regular diet on a special occasion can be thought of as a celebration, not a failure: a celebration of the birthday and of your spouse's recovery. It is okay to stop, experience your gratitude, and celebrate. And after such a break, you both can return to your heart-healthy food plan with renewed commitment.

3. Study the implications of your beliefs. What is the likelihood of a negative result in the event that your negative belief is correct? The question to ask is: Even if my belief is correct, what does that really imply?

When you look at the evidence, you may find it true that eating chocolate cake and ice cream caused your mate to exceed his daily fat gram goal and possibly gain a pound or two. The facts don't necessarily imply, however, that he is irresponsible, lacks willpower, or has permanently failed at his heart-healthy food plan. The real implications may be that your spouse is simply human and that occasional but temporary setbacks will occur.

4. Reflect on the usefulness of your beliefs. Judge the consequences of holding a particular belief, even if it is true. The question to ask yourself is: Is the belief destructive? Even if the belief is true now, is the situation changeable? And if it is changeable, how can I change it? Dwelling on the negative belief doesn't resolve anything. By focusing on what you can do and looking for solutions, you are more likely to achieve a sense of control and feel more positive about the future.

Right now your spouse may lack the necessary willpower to succeed with the heart-healthy food plan. Rather than give up on the plan or, more importantly, on your spouse, focus on methods he can use to strengthen his willpower and his commitment to the plan.

Bette and Dan illustrate the importance of learning to think positively. Bette came home unexpectedly and found Dan smoking in the garage. In a flash, her thoughts flew to her most catastrophic explanation. He didn't love her! He would rather smoke cigarettes and die than live to grow old with her. She accused him of total irresponsibility. She called him names and stalked out of the garage. Bette was determined never to discuss what had happened with Dan. She was furious and felt betrayed.

The incident might have ended in a stalemate, with Bette alienated from Dan and no resolution in sight. Using her new thinking techniques, Bette came to see things differently. It was irresponsible for Dan to be smoking because of his cardiac condition and rehabilitation program, but Bette's assumption of total irresponsibility was a catastrophic exaggeration. Dan was managing his food plan reasonably well, and was devout about his cardiovascular exercise. It was serious that Dan lied about having quit smoking, but Bette's assumption that everything Dan said was a lie kept her feeling hurt and hopeless.[6] By recognizing her feelings and using her optimistic thinking tools, Bette decided to discuss the situation with Dan. Communication opened between them, and together they laid the groundwork for further discussion and for a plan to support Dan in his difficult struggle to quit smoking.

Five Guidelines for Decision Making

In any crisis it's hard to think, but you face an additional pressure: the difficult task of making immediate life-or-death decisions—alone. Heartmates, who usually share the responsibility for making family decisions, now must do so without the support and input from their mates. There are pressing medical decisions to be made. At the onset of the crisis, when your mind is least functional, you are forced to act quickly and decisively.

Just hours after her husband's bypass surgery, as she was about to leave for home to get some much-needed rest, Helene was approached by her husband's medical team for permission to perform further surgery. Dennis was experiencing unexpected internal bleeding. Overwhelmed by a sense of responsibility for his life, Helene could barely think, much less make one more decision. Through her blur of exhaustion, she summoned what was left of her energy and signed the papers.

> While it may be necessary to make decisions about matters requiring immediate attention, limit your decision making during a crisis.

Premature decisions can be costly. Leave as many decisions as possible until you are better equipped to make them. Limiting your decision making will also reduce the stress and shock that you, the patient, and family are already suffering.

After Bill's wife, Carole, suffered a cardiac arrest and a stroke at age fifty-nine, they were advised that she would need to spend the rest of her life in a nursing home. Bill was horrified at the idea but too distraught to protest. Like a robot, he filled out the admittance forms. Carole was transferred from the hospital to the nursing home. Ten days later, she was literally climbing over the sides of her bed to use the bathroom. By this time, Bill had his wits about him. He and Carole decided that she should move back home. He would arrange for the assistance of a home health nurse, and she would participate in an intensive rehabilitation program.

Whether you must make snap decisions or you have time to consider your options, the choices you make will be better if your decision-making process is thoughtful and organized. I have reduced the process into five components to make it simpler, less overwhelming. Consider the five elements below as a guide to inform your decision making.

1. Prioritize. How important is the decision?
2. Involve others. Is this a decision to be made alone or with others?
3. Assess urgency. How urgent is the decision?
4. Weigh action vs. inaction. Does this decision require action?

5. Align decisions with values. What is the goal of this decision?
   Is it in line with my beliefs?

Prioritize

It is vital that you determine if a decision is urgent or if it can wait. Your energy is limited, and you are more likely to spin your wheels if you don't clarify your priorities. Once you decide that a decision is significant and pressing, you can concentrate your attention on it. You can free your mind of the burden of matters that can wait.

You can't do it all, so you'll need to establish priorities. Ask yourself how important the issue is to you, your spouse, your family. Will it have a long-term effect on your future, or is it something that will soon be forgotten? How much does it concern you? If making a medical decision is consistently on your mind, take care of it before moving on to other things. If lifestyle issues are most confusing, give them your attention.

Of course, when you are upset, fatigued, and confused, it isn't always obvious what should have your attention. How will you decide whether to do spring cleaning, weed your garden, attend a dinner party, participate in a college planning meeting with your high school senior, or walk three miles with your spouse?

What you really need is perspective. After you've asked yourself questions to assess and clarify your priorities, ask a trusted friend to look at a list of decisions that you think you should make. A fresh perspective may help you to see more clearly. Based on the intensity of your concern, long-range consequences, and a reality check, prioritize your decisions and deal with them one at a time as peacefully as possible.

Involve Others

Making decisions alone or cooperatively is a matter of individual style. In a crisis, people usually fall back on what is most familiar. The old way of doing things, however, may not be the best prescription for the situation at hand.

It is not uncommon for heartmates to assume full responsibility for decision making. They exclude their spouses, other family members, medical staff, or trusted friends who could offer suggestions and provide other perspectives. Certain decisions seem too trivial or too stressful to bother others with. As the partner and caregiver, it seems reasonable to handle everything alone.

On the other hand, because of the stress and intense pressure that accompany a cardiac event, many heartmates feel paralyzed in their ability to make decisions on their own. These heartmates tend to seek advice and counsel on most issues requiring a decision.

Assuming full control can be isolating, yet only seeking answers from others will sabotage your self-esteem and make you feel incompetent and dependent. Strive for a balance. Assess the decisions you need to make and consider whether collaboration is necessary and beneficial or whether it would be better to make the decision on your own. Doing so will help you think more clearly, involve your partner and family in matters that directly concern them, and free you from the paralysis of indecision.

Assess Urgency

Timing is yet another serious element in decision making. There are decisions that need to be made in the moment, and there are others for which you have plenty of time to plan. Maintaining clarity can be tricky. In a crisis, your sense of time becomes distorted. Time can seem to stretch out to infinity when you're waiting to hear how your spouse has come through a surgical procedure. Or a long time can pass in the flash of a millisecond when you picture your years together before the cardiac crisis. When you are making a decision, it is important to put time and urgency into perspective.

*B*arely *two months after my husband's recovery from a second mild heart attack, his cardiologist suggested that he have an angiogram. His opinion afterward: "No surgery indicated; proceed with conservative treatment, including diet, exercise, and medication."*

Thoroughly frightened by two heart attacks, we sought a second opinion. The second cardiologist advised the exact opposite, saying, "If I were you, I'd have surgery as soon as possible." We were stunned! It never dawned on us that getting a second opinion would complicate our decision. We'd naively expected the second opinion to reassure us by verifying that the first cardiologist was "right." We had hoped to enhance our sense of safety. Instead, our anxiety tripled.

Our purpose was clear. We were committed to doing whatever would be best for my husband's health. But what was best? We struggled with the decision for a week, going over the advantages and disadvantages in our minds. Finally, we decided to accept the more conservative treatment: no bypass surgery. Just making a decision helped reduce our anxiety and stress.

Almost two years passed before circumstances changed radically. One morning, severe chest pains awakened my husband. The cardiologist scheduled an angiogram. Now our decision was urgent: his life was on the line. This time the choice was for surgery. Although we were scared about the surgery and disappointed that it was necessary, we were satisfied that we made the right choice.

Weigh Action vs. Inaction

Most people think of decision making as exclusively active, taking a stand or doing something. In fact, decision making often involves acceptance and trust, and being receptive to someone else's judgment. Accepting that there is nothing to be done is actually doing something. A decision not to act, not to schedule bypass surgery after my husband's two heart attacks, was as much of a decision as choosing to do so two years later.

Every decision you make is simultaneously saying yes to something and no to something else. Every yes is also no. We generally ignore the no because it implies loss and may be uncomfortable or unpleasant. Our conservative decision to go with medication, exercise, and a heart-healthy diet, for example, required that we say no to surgery. Whether your decision requires action or inaction, be positively involved in the process. Remember, there is almost never a "right" answer. Making a good decision means initiating action when it is appropriate and remaining still when that will be most beneficial. Accepting inaction in the face of danger requires courage and faith. There's little in life that is more demanding than simply waiting and being receptive to what comes.

Align Decisions with Your Values

Your values form the natural foundation for every decision you make. To establish the purpose of a decision, you will have to ask the question, "Why?" Struggling with this difficult question may not yield a specific answer, but it will help you formulate and articulate your goals. The reason for your decision might be general, such as expressing the love that you feel for your spouse, or specific, such as understanding and supporting a new exercise regimen.

Bernice, a talented and respected counselor, became a heartmate just after her fiftieth birthday. About six months after her husband's heart attack, she asked me to help her with a career decision. Bernice and Bernard's financial situation was secure. He had a solid offer to sell his small business and had decided, at age fifty-three, to retire early.

Until Bernard's heart attack, their marriage had been satisfying, but secondary. With two full-time careers and no children, they were both accustomed to being independent and going their own way. Bernard's illness brought them closer together. Bernice discovered that her husband meant more to her than she had ever thought. Confronted with the possibility of losing him, she realized that she wanted to make their relationship a higher priority in her life.

Bernice's goal was to reorganize her time so that it matched her newly discovered values. She tried to weigh the pros and cons of keeping or giving up her career. Retiring would mean that she and Bernard would have more time together. They would be able to relax, spend time quietly at the shore, and escape the stress of city life.

On the surface, it seemed like a perfect solution. Her family had never been supportive of her need for a career; it had always been a disappointment to them that Bernice hadn't chosen to be a homemaker and mother. On the other hand, her work was central to what made her feel valued. Having her own earned income, although it was much smaller than Bernard's, enhanced her independence and self-esteem. Without her job, she felt she would be giving up the only thing that she could call her own.

As she reexamined her priorities, Bernice realized how much she valued her marriage *and* her career. Both emerged as powerful rivals for first place on her list of priorities, so she chose a compromise aligned with her dual purpose of honoring herself and her relationship with Bernard. She elected to compress her working days to Tuesdays, Wednesdays, and Thursdays, an arrangement that freed up the rest of her week to spend with Bernard. Staying in touch with her values and sense of purpose helped Bernice turn an "either/or" decision into a "both/and" opportunity.

Making decisions that align your purpose with your values is difficult, particularly during the acute phase of a crisis, but also as you reorient your life during recovery. Crisis often demands that you reassess values you've long taken for granted, but rarely does it supply easy answers.

Major decisions require investigation and understanding followed by realignment of your actions in harmony with carefully considered values. These values bear the weight of familial, ethnic, cultural, and religious beliefs. Taking time to think about your decisions can keep you anchored to the values and purpose that are the foundation of your actions. Commit your considerations to paper. Writing can help you stay on track. Here is a guide for processing decision making.

HEARTMATES® GUIDE FOR DECISION MAKING

- What is the decision I face? (State it as clearly.)
- What is my purpose for making this decision?
- What options are open to me that will help me achieve my purpose? (List all options you can think of, including those you know you would not ultimately choose.)
- What are the positives and negatives (the costs) of each option? What will be the result or consequence of each option? To me? To my spouse? To our family? To others?
- What feelings do I have as I deliberate about this decision? How much weight should I give them in considering my decision?

- Are there things I need to know, to learn about, before I can finalize this decision? How can I get the information I need?
- Now that I have considered these questions, I will make a decision and commit it to writing: "I have decided to . . ."or "I choose to. . . ."
- How do I feel about having made this decision? Is ambivalence or another feeling getting in the way of acting on my choice?
- I won't avoid necessary decisions. Not deciding is a decision.
- I will remember my original purpose as I act on my decision.
- I will celebrate my success!

Directing Communications: Decisions, Decisions

Director of communications is a title automatically conferred on you as mate and partner, and your task is to manage the information clearinghouse. Your access to the patient makes you the obvious source of information for family and friends. You are expected to provide medical reports and relay messages to the patient. Everyone means well and sends love and best wishes. Their support is appreciated, but it's exhausting to repeat every detail of recovery each time someone calls.

Director of communications is a role that requires a clear head and a great deal of decision making. Everyone: his parents, his children, your children, your parents, friends, his boss, and his coworkers must be informed. You need to consider carefully when and what to tell others. There just isn't any way to soften bad news. Although some cases are pretty straightforward, others are more sensitive. You wish you had a press secretary so the information could be passed more efficiently.

My most delicate call was to my husband's mother. Who would be more worried than his mother? Widowed twenty years earlier when her husband died after a heart attack, she, too, has heart disease. I was afraid that the shock might aggravate her condition.

I had to be careful about when to call (certainly not at midnight when he was diagnosed). Luckily, his condition was not so critical that I couldn't wait for morning. Then, there was the question of how much to say. At that point I hadn't seen any test results nor heard a prognosis. I wanted to give her an accurate picture without alarming her unnecessarily.

Complexities in family relationships predate the cardiac crisis. This can make communicating the seriousness of the situation an extremely complicated task. Remember, too, that family members' personal needs may override their consideration about what's best for your spouse's healing. Your words may be a balm for mending estranged relationships, or they may exacerbate an unhealthy situation, driving relatives apart. The further away family members are in miles and the more emotionally distant they are from your immediate family, the more helpless they will feel. They may even want you to take responsibility for their decisions, like whether they should come to visit.

> Don't expect yourself to shoulder responsibility for anyone beyond yourself and your partner. You are in no condition to take on the whole family and its history.

Your mate may want to see some relatives but not others. You are the designated spokesperson in the unenviable, uncomfortable position of having to say yes or no. You need to be tactful, but remember that your priority in this situation is to respect your spouse's needs.

If your children are grown and away, you will want to consider seriously and carefully whether *you* want them to come home. You are entitled to express your preference. But they have the right to want to come home. You need to weigh the emotional benefits of their presence against the potential disruption in all of your lives. How can you keep yourself from feeling as if you have to take care of them, too? Will you be loving and supportive to each other, or will old family conflicts flare up and cause additional stress?

One man thought twice before calling their son during his college exams to inform him that his mother had suffered a heart attack. Another heartmate made the decision, with her fingers crossed, not to send for their two daughters, who were at music camp. Still another knew instinctively that their thirty-year-old daughter wouldn't rest easy until she saw her father with her own two eyes.

Some patients are adamant about not wanting anyone but you at the hospital. Some parents don't want to "bother the children" or have them "see Dad this way." For some families, especially those with children or grandchildren, it may be wise to put off visitors until the patient has returned home from the hospital, is feeling less vulnerable, and is "on the mend." Others are comforted by having the whole family gathered around from the onset of the crisis.

It's hard to think about everyone else's needs when you can barely get your own head on straight. Matters can be further complicated. You may be asked indirectly whether you think your mate will survive. You may not be prepared or willing to confront this question. Children may ask directly, "Is my Dad going to die?" Is there a way to provide an honest and realistic answer and still manage to comfort a young child? What is good counsel for your grown son, who is trying to make a decision about leaving his own family in another part of the country to be with his parents?

You cannot always make wise decisions when you are dealing with an unknown and uncertain future. What if your mate doesn't survive? Would it be better or worse if the children were present? What are the psychological risks if they aren't there and their parent dies? There are no easy answers.

Practice your decision-making skills, and don't let other people's urgency and fear pressure you. You may be too upset or exhausted to make any decisions except those that are absolutely critical. You can prioritize your decisions. You can't predict the future. "I don't know" is a perfectly acceptable answer. *You're not responsible for knowing everything or taking care of everyone.*

Considering the Deeper Questions

The cardiac crisis brings you face to face with how much control you really have. Sometimes, no matter how well-informed or decisive you are, there are areas over which you have little or no control or authority. You can't make heart disease disappear. You can't change what has already happened to you and your mate because of heart disease. You can't even change how you feel about it.

Your power is limited to choosing your attitude about what is happening. You can be in charge of the way you will accept and adapt to a new reality, a new life.

The Whisper That Guides

Living with unanswerable questions ranges from emotionally uncomfortable to agonizing. It is a rare individual who would choose uncertainty over security. But accepting your powerlessness also has its rewards.

Your day-to-day life has been ruptured by a cardiac crisis. All your perceptions are altered. The result can be an awakening to a deeper level of thinking and coping with your feelings. You may experience it as a sense that something is different, has shifted. You may have a momentary flash that "life is not forever" or that "this relationship is precious." Many cardiac spouses do not recognize these flashes, because the everyday mind is so insistent and demanding. But those who have this revelation describe it as a whisper rising in the rare moments when the mind calms down.

The whisper directs you to the deeper questions that are an integral, though often buried, part of the cardiac crisis. These questions invite you to explore issues beyond medications, diets, and daily routines. They provoke serious thought about mortality, purpose, the meaning of your relationships, your life. They ask you to look at yourself in relation to the larger world, to other heartmates, to all people in pain, and even to all others on our planet.

Sure, it's easier to stay involved with the practical questions; the unknown can be excruciating. Many cardiac spouses may have conscientiously avoided such questions since childhood or adolescence. Others have outgrown the answers they accepted then, but haven't had the occasion to reexamine them until now. Still others may be disillusioned by the idealistic answers of youth. It is natural to push nagging questions away by saying, "None of this really matters," or, "I haven't got time to think about this. I have to take care of the everyday tasks that fill my life," or, like Scarlett O'Hara, to promise yourself to think about it . . . tomorrow.

The everyday part of the mind clamors, scrambling for concrete answers; it loves cholesterol levels and milligrams, the countable, the measurable, and the knowable. The whispering question doesn't seek the right answer; it only needs permission to be heard. Simply contemplating issues and struggling to understand questions will move you along your path of meaning, your spiritual path.

> Recovery is an ideal time to ponder the realm of
> meaning and purpose.

The cardiac crisis has made you vulnerable, and you are more likely to see the gravity of those deeper questions about the meaning and quality of your life. The protection of normal, daily life and the illusions of being powerful and in full control have broken down. In a time of crisis, the whisper can be heard.

Should you choose to listen for and respond to that whisper, give yourself some regular quiet time. Find a place where you can think undisturbed; go for a walk, take a long, hot bath, or sit in your favorite easy chair. Be gentle and patient with yourself. Start a diary or a journal to keep an ongoing record of your experience for later reflection.[7] Or pursue your thoughts and questions by sharing them with a trusted friend, a mentor, or a spiritual guide. There is no "right" way to ponder the deeper questions. Whatever your individual style, take advantage of the opportunity.

SOME THOUGHTS ON THINKING

- Limited concentration and the inability to focus are normal responses to a cardiac crisis.
- Thinking patterns return to normal more slowly than feelings.
- Reviewing the events of your cardiac story is a natural and healing mental response.
- Repetition can transform chaos and confusion into a sense of order and meaning.
- Recognizing feelings is a first step to untangling thoughts.
- Sharing thoughts can give you another's perspective and a valuable reality check.
- Postpone unnecessary decision making whenever possible until you have more control over your thinking.
- The everyday, rational part of your mind is an important resource in decision making.
- The quiet, abstract part of your mind connects you to questions of meaning and to your internal wisdom.

Chapter 4 Notes

1. Rhoda F. Levin, "Life Review: A Natural Process," in *Readings in Psychosynthesis: Theory, Process, and Practice* (Toronto: Ontario Institute for Studies in Education, 1985), 82–96.
2. William Bridges, *Transitions: Making Sense of Life's Changes* (Reading, Mass.: Addison-Wesley, 1980): a supportive and readable study about the journey of change, and how to accept it and grow from it.

3. Discussion of reactions to trauma in *Trauma and Recovery* by Judith Herman, MD, (New York: Basic Books, 1997), 34: "Fragmentation, whereby trauma tears apart a complex system of self-protection that normally functions in an integrated fashion, is central to the historic observations on post-traumatic stress disorder. . . ." On page 45, Herman relates her phrase "paralysis of the mind" to Robert Jay Lifton's "psychic numbing," which he coined in his renowned studies of survivors of disaster and war.

Judith Herman, MD, proposes effective preventive education when people like heartmates have suffered from a recent acute trauma, the cardiac event. She proposes the following: 1) patient, mate, family, and friends should be given clear, detailed information regarding post-traumatic reactions so that they are less frightening when they occur; 2) patient, mate, family, and friends should be prepared for disruptions in relationships that normally follow a traumatic experience so that they can be tolerant and take these disruptions in stride; and 3) patient, mate, and family should be given advice on coping strategies and warned about common mistakes so that their sense of competence and efficacy will not suffer.

4. Contact Aging with Dignity, whose user-friendly project "Five Wishes" helps people think through, write, and accomplish the legalities necessary to provide for end-of-life care and for dying. Contact them for your copy of this pamphlet: P.O. Box 1661, Tallahassee, Florida 32302, (850) 681-2010, or <www.agingwithdignity.org>.

Explore the concept of creating a document to leave your legacy to loved ones. Visit <www.womenslegacies.com> for information about *Women's Lives, Women's Legacies: Passing Your Beliefs and Blessings to Future Generations* (Minneapolis: Fairview Press, 2003), by Rachael Freed. Other resources include *Ethical Wills: Putting Your Values on Paper,* by Barry K. Baines, MD (New York: Perseus, 2001), and the Legacy Center at <www.thelegacycenter.net>.

5. Martin E. P. Seligman, PhD, *Learned Optimism* (New York: Alfred A. Knopf, 1990), 221–25. This important book presents a powerful argument and practical techniques for overcoming pessimistic thinking.

Personal control is the opposite of helplessness; it indicates the ability to think about, decide, and take personal action to change things. Most of us mistakenly believe that it is control over feelings that makes us less helpless.

It has been statistically shown that the more changes (stressors) a person encounters in a period of time, the greater the risk for depression and illness, including heart attacks and cancer. Factors or stressors that affect health include loss, pessimism, depression, catecholamine depletion, endorphin depletion, immune suppression, and disease (Seligman, 182).

The other major factor defining risk for illness and prediction for recovery is social support. The capacity to love and sustain meaningful friendships, as opposed to being friendless and isolated, can be a marker for recovery.

For those interested in the topic of changing negative thinking, I also recommend John Roger and Peter McWilliams' book, *You Can't Afford the Luxury of a Negative Thought* (Los Angeles: Prelude Press, 1988).

6. Mary Hayes-Grieco calls hope a discipline, not a feeling, in her book, *The Kitchen Mystic: Spiritual Lessons Hidden in Everyday Life* (Center City, Minn.: Hazelden Books, 1992). "Hope is a set of behaviors and attitudes you adopt to carry you forward as if your life matters, even though at the moment you may feel that it doesn't. When you are facing a time of emotion and lack of direction, it is an act of hope to tend to health habits like eating and sleeping and to keep a minimum level of beauty and order in your appearance and environment."

7. Journaling can be an aid in clarifying thoughts and reflecting on loss. A useful resource for journaling is Julia Cameron's book, *The Artist's Way* (New York: Tarcher, 1992). Don't be put off by the word "artist." This book is the ultimate self-care book, based on Twelve-Step wisdom. I have been journaling the recommended three pages daily for many years. It is the best self-care, healing, and spiritual discipline for me. I'm not the only one. This book has been a best-seller for years. You can find journaling groups and classes, in most communities, that use the techniques in this book.

I also recommend the *The Heartmates Journal: A Companion for Partners of People with Serious Illness* (Minneapolis: Fairview Press, 2002). This is a year-long recovery journal with weekly readings and quotations; questions to guide journal writing; blank pages for journaling; and suggested qualities, such as compassion or creativity, to focus your reflection.

5

Shifting Responsibility: From Caretaker to Partner

You led an active, full life before the cardiac crisis. Whether at home, in your special relationships, or in your career, you handled the daily demands of your life. You probably weren't looking for any extra work or stress.

But from the moment your mate became a cardiac patient, your responsibilities changed. Regardless of the division of labor prior to the cardiac event, you are now saddled with both your share *and* your mate's.

The Scenario: Changing Responsibilities

In the acute stage of the crisis, your responsibilities simply snowballed. Suddenly, you were in charge of medical decisions, financial arrangements, and the emotional needs of your family. Your mate was bedridden and, for a time, maybe unable even to speak. His only responsibility was to rest so that his heart would heal. You were responsible for *everything* else.

The dramatic switch in responsibility is intensified because you are in crisis, too. Your anxiety is heightened and even simple decisions seem overwhelming. Normal demands seem heavier and less manageable. And the crisis creates new jobs and still more responsibilities as you keep family and friends informed, while running the household single-handedly.

Once your mate returns home, your hands are full in other ways. Because hospital stays are usually short, you end up supplying your mate with semiskilled nursing care. Your spouse's physical activity is limited, and he may spend much time resting. The majority of your time is spent preparing and serving meals, changing bedding, and monitoring medications. Tack on your roles as communications director and chief decision maker, and it quickly becomes clear that you've been asked to accept more than a handful of responsibility.

Most of us look forward to the end of hospitalization, but we can't anticipate the complexity of the situation that follows. Expecting that homecoming will simply be a joyous celebration is unrealistic.

> The end of the hospital stay is both a joyful celebration and the beginning of a complex phase of recovery.

You may have imagined that everything would return to normal, to the way it was before the cardiac event, but that's not the case. As wonderful as it is to have your mate home, everything is different. Established patterns and daily routines have been disrupted and redefined. A new chain of command excluding the patient has developed within the family. You may feel discouraged or resentful about being questioned or second-guessed for decisions made during hospitalization.

You may be surprised to find yourself riding an emotional roller coaster. One minute you're overjoyed, the next disappointed and confused. This is the beginning of an ongoing period of recovery. It's normal to have mixed feelings as you, the patient, and your family strive to understand and accept circumstances and situations that continue to change.

Family dynamics will never return to your idealized memory of "normal," to the way they were before heart disease. You all struggle to make sense of the event and the changes it continues to demand. Heart disease can happen in any family. It happens in families that are resilient and strong and in those for whom heart disease feels like the "last straw" amid preexisting chaos. Unresolved family issues, such as alcoholism, codependency, abuse, or chronic unemployment, can heighten the stress and difficulty of adjusting to heart disease.

Patients, clearly, have been deeply affected by the cardiac event and are confronted with their own issues. Much of their energy is consumed, consciously or unconsciously, in confronting their own mortality. Some patients return home to find their power in the household and their responsibility for discipline of children usurped by their well spouse. Others come home weak and unsure about their health and future, and they feel like their dependence on spouse and children makes them a burden to the family. Still others feel replaced and unneeded if their spouse and children have become more independent.

As if your immediate family's dynamics were not demanding enough, it is incumbent on you to make sure that friends and relatives don't overstay their visits. You feel it's up to you to make sure that your mate doesn't get overly taxed or exhausted. And, despite your own fatigue, you may feel obliged to play hostess by taking reservations for visiting hours, serving coffee and sweets, and cleaning up after the guests are gone. Entertaining adds to your stress when you are coping with a crisis. Although some visitors are a source of comfort and you welcome them with open arms, others can be more of a hindrance than help.

As the recovery phase progresses, new responsibilities emerge. Even if your mate is recovering relatively smoothly, you still spend hours catering heart-healthy meals and driving him to appointments. Some cardiac patients are depressed and, by default, may leave the majority of daily responsibilities to you. Months down the road, you may find yourself stuck, unable to stop caretaking. If your spouse faces early retirement, you may be financially pressured to assume the role of sole breadwinner and caretaker. Running back and forth between job and home responsibilities can only add more anxiety and stress.

Shifting responsibility is one of the most complex issues you face. On the surface, choices seem obvious: Your mate needs help, so it's natural for you to assume the responsibility. And the fact that he's depending on you makes you want to rise to the occasion.

Because of the unexpected and sudden onset of the crisis, you simply take on whatever needs to be done. You may believe that you have no choice and that loving your spouse means picking up all the slack.

> You can measure the level of responsibility you assume by observing how you spend your time every day.

Understanding your patterns of responsibility and how much you and your mate depend on each other, however, is more complicated. Patterns that took years to develop are firmly entrenched in your relationship. Caring for your sick spouse either cements existing patterns, or creates entirely new ones.

You may be aware of accepting major responsibilities, but there are probably many others that you have assumed unconsciously. Whether or not you are aware of them, these new patterns reshape the foundation of your relationship. Habits establish themselves quickly. Temporary emergency measures quickly evolve into a permanent change in the division of labor.

Some heartmates thrive on crisis, pressure, and responsibility. If you're this kind of person, you might welcome the opportunity to take charge. Other heartmates find crisis and recovery wearisome. All heartmates, however, experience times of feeling overwhelmed, frustrated, and resentful. All of these responses are normal.

> Be aware of your feelings. This will prepare you to examine the progress of your recovery, appraise your relationship, and take care of yourself.

Identifying and understanding changes in responsibility herald the beginning of your recovery. You begin to take better care of yourself, clarifying and managing your responsibilities as well as the feelings that go with them.

Consider taking the following questionnaire to examine your responsibilities. Begin by evaluating those you had before the cardiac event. Then, look at the responsibilities you've taken on since.

HEARTMATES® RESPONSIBILITY QUESTIONNAIRE

Pre-cardiac Crisis

1. Which spouse took more responsibility in each of the following areas:
    income
    family finances
    meals
    housework
    yard work
    parenting children (yours together, his, yours)
    relationships with grown children (yours together, his, yours)
    caring for aging parents (his, yours)
    social and recreational activities
    your relationship with each other
    spiritual life

2. In what ways was your spouse dependent on you?

3. In what ways were you dependent on your spouse?

4. Have the two of you become more or less dependent on each other throughout the life of your relationship?

5. Did you consider yourself:
      independent
      too independent
      dependent
      too dependent
      interdependent
      responsible
      overresponsible
      underresponsible

Post-cardiac Crisis

1. Which responsibilities have changed? What do you do
   now that's different? How do you feel about your new
   responsibilities?

2. How are you more dependent on your spouse now?

3. How are you less dependent on your spouse now?

4. How is your spouse more dependent on you now?

5. How is your spouse less dependent on you now?

By assuming your responsibilities as a heartmate, you deserve respect
and recognition from your mate, family, friends—and yourself. And
yet you may be tempted to tolerate inconvenience, incessant
demands, and unrelenting pressure. Challenge your feelings of guilt
and obligation.

> Manage your responsibilities. Delegate those you
> can and set limits to those you cannot. You are
> important, too, as are your needs and
> limitations.

Responsibility and Love

It is natural and appropriate to assume more responsibility during a crisis. There is nothing more disturbing than seeing someone you love helpless and suffering. You want to do anything and everything you can to help. Heartmates should be awarded a Purple Heart for bravery. Your genuine love and concern for your partner is expressed when you take charge in a loving and compassionate way.

After bypass surgery, my husband was moved to the intensive care unit. I was thoroughly unprepared for what I witnessed when I first saw him there. Under the huge overhead heating lamp, and attached to several strange-sounding machines and a respirator, he looked like an alien from outer space. He lay very still and his skin felt cold and stiff. He was barely awake and had a morphine drip for pain.

He had been invaded—to his very core. A half dozen tubes he could not control led into and out of his body. Even his nose and throat had tubes running into them, making it impossible for him to speak. He had no way to let me know that his lips were dry, that he'd appreciate something cool and wet. He had no way to express his fear, anger, or pain. He had no way to celebrate the fact that he was alive.

I felt immense compassion for him. I chose to be his protection, his shield. I committed myself to being the buffer between his total vulnerability and the outside world.

We quickly devised a communication system. He wrote out his questions, tracing one letter at a time with his finger on the sheet at his side. I read his tracing aloud, and when I was correct, he would move on. If not, he would indicate my mistake by raising his index finger, and repeat the letter again. It was a slow process. Sometimes he would forget in the middle of spelling a word and slide into a morphine snooze. (Magic Slates or small dry-erase boards should be standard equipment in cardiac care units.)

The first question he traced on the sheet was "What time is it?" I looked at my watch and told him it was 4:30. He became very upset. He began tracing again. "W-H-A-T D-A-Y?" I began to understand how lost, how helpless, how vulnerable he was. He didn't even know what day it was or how long he had been there. It had been a long and difficult day for me, too, but I vowed to stand there until I couldn't stand anymore, to do what I could for my mate.

Later one of the machines made a new noise, beeped a different message. Asked to step out of the unit, I returned to find my husband agitated. Back to the sheet and the tracing. One letter at a time, but I got the picture. He'd tried to ask the nurse why the machine was making the noise. Her response: "Don't worry about it; you're doing fine." If she'd intended to reassure him, she succeeded in accomplishing the opposite. Being patronized only aggravated him.

When the nurse returned, I said I wanted to know about the sound. She explained that the machine was reporting a malfunction. Within minutes, the machine was replaced with another that beeped like a familiar friend.

I was my husband's shield, his voice, his protection. It was necessary . . . and satisfying. The next morning the tubes were removed from his throat, and he COULD speak for himself.

As soon as he could talk, my speaking for him became an insult. When patients are just out of surgery, or have just suffered a heart attack, they require total care, like newborn children. But just as children gradually become more independent, cardiac patients rapidly advance to independence. A parent who does too much for a youngster fosters dependence and handicaps the child.

> At each stage of recovery, it's crucial for heartmates to determine what their mates can and can't handle. Relinquish responsibility accordingly.

You might be genuinely pleased to see your mate gradually resuming care of his own needs. His increased involvement is a positive sign of recovery. Or you might experience some ambivalence. Just as some parents find it hard to let go, you might feel hesitant about stepping back and letting your spouse fend for himself.

Supporting your mate's recovery means noticing and encouraging his efforts toward independence. But after witnessing your spouse's utter helplessness in the hospital, how can you help being overly protective? While you're understandably worried that he might do too much and relapse, don't let your fear stand in the way of his recovery.

Heartmates can have trouble shifting gears and discovering how much their partners can realistically handle. One heartmate insisted on spoon-feeding her husband even though he had been eating without assistance the day following surgery. Another heartmate imposed mandatory rest periods, even when her husband wasn't tired. Heartmates often misunderstand the medical warning to avoid stress. They "take over" to protect their partners from the danger of any and all stress. One forbade her husband to watch the news on TV.

> Modify your caretaking to match your mate's progress.

Don't do everything for him, only your appropriate share. To help yourself assess and let go of old caretaking responsibilities, review your image of your mate as a patient and reassess his physical progress. As he becomes stronger, work at changing your image of yourself, too—from heroine to helpmate. Remember that medical professionals have a graduated, step-by-step plan to wean heart patients from total care. You can feel confident that he is well enough to do things for himself and function without round-the-clock care.

If you find that you are afraid to stop overprotecting your mate, you're not alone. To help wean heartmates from the patients' bedsides, one progressive hospital provides each spouse with a beeper for the duration of the patient's stay. The beeper functions as a symbol of recognition of the spouse. Only people important in the recovery process have beepers. Beepers also serve as self-care tools, freeing heartmates to take better care of themselves during the acute crisis. They can roam the hospital, take a walk in the fresh air, or even go home for a much-needed nap, always remaining in instantaneous contact with the hospital staff.[1]

For your spouse to maintain the role of patient or "victim" is emotionally destructive and will actually slow physical recovery.

Encouraging your mate to remain helpless isn't healthy for either of you. *Both of you are in a period of recovery.* While your efforts to help are clearly motivated by caring and concern, taking on too much responsibility may ultimately backfire, trapping you and him. A combination of rest and some responsibility is the best way for your mate to regain strength and confidence.

> Your recovery also depends on managing an ongoing shift in the balance of power and responsibility. This management leads you to discover "right responsibility."

Responsibility and Fear

Right responsibility is supportive and loving. However, in a crisis, there is the risk of assuming too much responsibility. In the context of a health crisis, right responsibility means basing your actions on an accurate perception of reality and striving for appropriate and balanced action and participation. Taking on more responsibility than is warranted is overresponsibility.

> Calling the rescue squad when your mate is having unremitting chest pain is perfectly appropriate. Calling the doctor every time your spouse looks pale, however, is an example of overresponsibility.

Fear is the number one cause of overresponsibility. Feelings are powerful, and fear is one of the most potent. The fear you experience may be out of proportion to the present situation, such as when you're convinced that your mate is on the verge of another heart attack, even though the physician just prescribed more physical activity and less medication. Heartmates entertain a wide range of exaggerated fears from losing sleep over one salty pretzel or fantasizing divorce after an angry outburst.

Your fears may go back to an earlier time when you felt as though you were in danger. When fear arises in the present, it can be intensified by memories of childhood, a time when you were more helpless and dependent. One of the most universal of all human fears is that of being abandoned. Nearly losing your mate almost always triggers this universal fear.

Intense fear blends with an all-consuming sense of responsibility to produce an awesome burden. The experience is something like bringing your first newborn home from the hospital. Everything revolves around a baby's schedule and demands. When you aren't actively caring for the baby, you worry if he or she is okay. You listen intently for sounds indicating that the baby is still alive after a nap or a night's sleep.

Your mate is *not* a totally helpless infant. And you are not completely vulnerable to your fear of losing your mate. Yet when your fear escalates, you may respond by acting overly responsible, staying awake through most of the night to check your mate's breathing, or waking him to ask if he took his medications.

It is important to note, however, that if your partner has chronic congestive heart failure, your recovery will involve a movement toward greater responsibility. As your mate becomes sicker, you will need to provide more and more care. Though difficult, it remains crucial for you to manage your fear and check yourself to ensure that you are not being overly responsible.

Listening for your partner's breathing is a perfectly normal reaction after all you've been through. But sacrificing your sleep in order to be the permanent night nurse is a sign of deeper, likely unfounded fears. When you find your fear overwhelming your sense of right responsibility, try the following techniques to reclaim your balance:

- Do deep breathing. Sit in a straight-backed chair with your feet on the floor. Focus on following your breath . . . in and out. Don't change your natural rhythm. Imagine that each time you inhale you breathe in calm and clarity. Each time you exhale you release fear and overresponsibility. Your body will be unable to hold on to intense fear as you concentrate on your breath. Continue focused breathing for one minute. Build up to five minutes.

- Use positive self-talk. Tell yourself that you have a choice about what you say to yourself, what you believe, how you interpret what is happening in your present situation. Here is the perfect opportunity to build and practice solid affirmations generated from your qualities of strength and courage. Affirmations should always be worded positively. Use your personal language style so you know that the affirmations are yours.

- Share with another person. You'll gain fellowship, social support, and perspective. What rolls around endlessly in your own mind continues to gather power. Overwhelming dark thoughts shrink to a controllable size when exposed to the light of day. Another person can serve as a reality check because he or she is not intimately affected by the situation as you are.

Survival Fear

Human beings have an emotional and psychological defense mechanism to protect them from enormous threats, from difficult and painful feelings. The psyche devises ways to function even in extreme fear. In order to function in your daily life, you may ignore, rationalize, or deny your fear. You are probably unaware of the extent of your fear on a day-to-day basis. But feelings left unaddressed do not go away and often "come out sideways."

If you're like most heartmates, your worst fear is that your mate will die. How terrifying to consider the possibility of losing your mate. Beneath this fear of loss is, perhaps, a deeper dread of being left alone: "Can I survive this loss? If my partner dies, how will I go on?" You've probably protected yourself against this fear. But whether or not you're aware of them, your fears about loss, abandonment, and your own survival manifest in a number of ways.

The heart-to-heart bond between you and your mate may become a conduit for unspoken fears. You reinforce and feed one another's fears, though each of your fears may be unique. You may be anxious about your mate coming home from the hospital, for example, sensing a greater risk now that he is no longer under the care of medical staff. You try to limit your mate's activities so he won't "overdo." Before you know it, he senses your insecurity and begins to question whether he's well enough to be at home. He starts checking his pulse several times a day and expects you to coddle him, convinced that he'd better not strain himself.

Fear of loss also makes loving couples turn away from much-needed physical affection. It's typical for cardiac couples to assume erroneously that sexual intercourse is too strenuous to be risked. Many couples pull back without discussion, each believing that he or she is protecting the other. Your recovering spouse may feel afraid of disappointing you by having less vitality or strength. And after everything you've been told about stressing the patient, it's difficult to relax and enjoy sexual activity.

> When you are ready to wean yourself from overre-sponsibility, you can begin by acknowledging and expressing your fears.

The worst of them is the fear of abandonment and that you won't survive the loss of your mate. Confronting and expressing your fears can help you begin to understand your overresponsibility. Face your fear with the belief that should the unspeakable happen, you will come out safely on the other side.

Search deep within yourself and affirm that you can survive. If you should lose your mate, it will be difficult, painful, and lonely, but few people actually die of broken hearts. Do your best to let go of the fear and return to living your life as fully as possible. Your mate's fears will more than likely diminish as he continues to recover. Fear may be intensified, not diminished, by neglecting intimacy. Physical intimacy can comfort and reassure both of you.

Too Much Dependence and Control

It's common for heart patients to express fear by becoming overly dependent on, or overly controlling of, their mates. There are patients, for example, who want their heartmates to be the only visitor at the hospital. Without even telling their partners why, these patients expect their mates to sit in a bedside vigil all day, with no relief from other visitors. And this behavior may continue once these patients return home.

John, an extremely busy account executive at a television station, took three weeks off from work when his wife had bypass surgery. Well into her recovery, his wife found reasons to keep John home, berating him whenever he left the house. Diane's frightened husband wouldn't grant her five minutes to do a load of laundry in the basement unless a close relative was nearby. Imagine her frustration over virtually being a prisoner in her own home. Under the grip of such fear and dependency, it becomes extremely difficult to tell where you end and your partner begins.

Patients are naturally preoccupied with their symptoms and emotions. Your mate may cope with his fear by being sullen, aggressive, or demanding in a desperate effort to regain control of his life. He may act like a prima donna, expecting you to wait on him hand and foot. And you may react by becoming even more focused on your spouse, lavishing extra attention on him, further adapting your lifestyle to his.

You may assume overresponsibility in a sincere but misguided effort to assist your spouse. You may put yourself in charge of risk factor control, carefully investigating ingredients in foods or becoming an outspoken advocate of nonsmoking.

One heartmate, Anita, believed every fad that advertised a magical elimination of heart disease, not realizing that her efforts to control made every meal a battleground. Gloria proudly described how she protected Milton from stress. She awakened before him, reviewed the morning newspaper, and cut out every article she decided was too distressing for him to read. (Were there even borders to hold on to when Milton opened his paper?) How could he feel competent, strong, and whole in relation to Gloria? How could Gloria feel free from the stress of her assumed burden?

Some cardiac spouses take on the role of peacemaker and censor all communication among family members in an effort to keep the household stress free. Others become increasingly isolated as they build a lifestyle centered around their mate's needs instead of their own.

These examples of over-dependency, control, and overresponsibility are like symptoms of addiction. The difference here is that the addiction is to a partner suffering from heart disease rather than to a chemical. An addict is a person whose well-being depends on an external source of support and security.[2] You and your mate may be unwittingly involved in an addictive relationship if he believes he needs you to take care of his every need and you believe that your identity and worth are solely dependent on providing his care. The longer this cycle continues, the harder it is to break and the more destructive it becomes to your relationship.

> Strive to give and receive in ways that are mutually helpful, appropriate, respectful, and empowering.

My fear that my husband would die and leave me led to overresponsible behavior that strained our relationship.

Once he was home from the hospital, I felt so afraid, so powerless to keep him alive, that I endowed his pills with that power. If he just took every pill, on time, everything would be okay. He would recover. He wouldn't have another heart attack. He wouldn't die.

I reminded him regularly about his medications. It became a routine part of my day to check that he'd taken his pills at the prescribed hour. The fact that he lived through each day was proof that my reminders were working. It never occurred to me that I was interfering. It never crossed my mind that he heard anything but my concern. I never imagined that he resented my questions.

One day, after listening to me go through my litany, my dear friend Shirley said, "He's a grown man, perfectly capable of monitoring his own medications. Stop nagging. It must be driving him crazy." I was so surprised. I hadn't heard myself nag. I thanked Shirley and went home to undo what, by then, had become habitual. It was excruciating for several days, like withdrawal from a drug. It took all my energy to keep quiet, to keep from saying, "Have you taken your pills?"

One morning I came across his pill box next to the bathroom sink. He had already left for his cardiac rehabilitation class and wouldn't return home until evening. I stood there paralyzed, wondering whether I should take his pills to him at his class or deliver them to his office. For a brief moment, I fantasized him having another heart attack. Surely if that happened it would be my fault. Then I saw how silly that was. I said to myself, "He can take care of himself; it isn't my responsibility." And suddenly the spell was broken. I was free!

I beat the meds, but the real issue was bigger: to break the pattern of dependency that had deepened with my husband's illness. I needed to deal with my fear, so that we could have an equal relationship based on mutual dignity and respect.

Returning home that evening, he asked me if I'd noticed that he'd forgotten his pills. I acknowledged seeing the box near the sink, and he said, "It's a good thing I keep an extra day's dose in my desk drawer at the office." He can take care of himself; he can handle the responsibility. I had been overreacting.

Unaddressed and unacknowledged fear is at the core of dependency and control. Fear motivates us to live outside of ourselves, to believe that we must abandon ourselves for a drug, a drink—or another person. When you let your fear get the best of you, the resulting dependency damages your sense of self and your relationships.

> Acknowledge your fears and examine your actions. If you feel you and your mate have an addictive, dependent relationship, start your "withdrawal program" today.

Recovery from dependency and control doesn't happen overnight or without effort, but you can do it.

Flexibility: Walking the Line

There can be a fine line between right responsibility and overresponsibility. Your mate, for example, may remain so incapacitated that you will need to handle or delegate most of the responsibilities. This is right responsibility. Your mate, alternatively, may progress in his recovery, becoming better able to take on responsibility himself.

> Assessment, priority setting, and flexibility are keys to sorting out appropriate responsibility.

Regardless of your partner's status, it's good to stop and evaluate the situation from time to time. How much is your mate able to do without your help? What responsibilities are urgent, and which can be set aside? What are the tasks that only you can take care of, and which can be shared by friends, relatives, or professional service providers?

One cardiac spouse, Rita, described her struggle with right responsibility and overresponsibility as a back-and-forth affair. Steve's first heart attack occurred twelve years ago. Just as he was getting back on his feet, he had a second heart attack. Recovery was slow, but Rita gradually resumed her own life, as Steve resumed responsibility for his own physical care. Then suddenly, after some years, Steve's condition deteriorated dramatically. After a third heart attack and congestive heart failure, he is often mentally confused and requires constant monitoring. Through no fault of her own, Rita is back to doling out medications and assuming responsibility for Steve's physical well-being. She is hungry for her freedom and anxious to give up the role of nurse. Their one ray of hope is that Steve is a heart-transplant candidate. In the meantime, Rita's responsibilities continue to shift from day to day.

It's natural to feel resentful when you have to assume an inordinate amount of responsibility, especially over a long period of time. You may feel sad or angry about the time and energy consumed in doing more than your share. And rightly so. If your mate's condition requires you to bear long-term responsibilities, allow yourself to feel the weight of the burden.[3]

> Pretending to be Superwoman or grumbling under your breath won't help you feel better or change your situation.

Try to remain flexible. Whatever your mate's health condition, continue reevaluating the situation. (See the Heartmates Responsibility Checklist below to help you with your assessment.) If you determine you are being overly responsible, find ways to right the balance. If you're practicing right responsibility but are still overwhelmed, seek assistance or take measures to alleviate your burden. When you combine flexibility with shared decision making, your taking on, shifting, or reassigning responsibilities can be a positive part of both your recovery and relationship.

HEARTMATES® RESPONSIBILITY CHECKLIST

Right Responsibility	Overresponsibility
Based on reality	An overreaction
Makes you feel calm	Makes you feel panicky
Well thought out	Urgent
Planned	Reckless
Comes from confidence	Motivated by fear
Allows for flexibility	Rigid and uncompromising

Stress: The Mysterious Threat

Stress, defined as a risk factor of heart disease, is often misunderstood and misdiagnosed. The word alone can send chills of terror up and down your spine. Early in the cardiac crisis, you're given the "Don't stress the patient" message. The warning is often interpreted as an injunction against sharing worries, concerns, and fears. You stifle your feelings, thinking that you are protecting your mate from stress. You may even take on your mate's worries, trying to reduce his stress load by increasing your own.

While cardiac patients are equally sensitive to and terrified of the stress myth, they sometimes use "stress" as an excuse to avoid uncomfortable situations. It isn't unusual to hear a cardiac patient blame or threaten a spouse with some variation of the statement, "Don't raise your voice; you'll make me have another heart attack." Or perhaps, more subtly, you get the message that to disagree with the patient is dangerous to his health. It isn't!

The term "stress" is used generically by many people, heartmates included, further complicating any firm understanding of what stress really is. "I need help coping with stress," is really a call for help in dealing with uncomfortable feelings or for finding appropriate avenues of expression or relief. Physical expression or activities that help people relax are often referred to as "stress reducers." Running, or any type of exercise, therapeutic massage, and warm baths are activities recommended to help the cardiac spouse and patient alike to reduce stress.

| Stress can be emotional as well as physical.

Are emotional and physical stress related? How can we tell the difference? It seems frustratingly clear that stress is a mystery.

What Is Stress, Really?
Dr. Robert Eliot's attempts to solve the mysteries of stress and its relationship to heart disease have been inconclusive. He maintains that while we know, or think we know, what stress is, each person experiences stress in a highly individual way.[4]

Four weeks after her heart attack, Julie felt frustrated because her doctor hadn't given her permission to drive her car. It was stressful to depend on someone else to chauffeur her around. But the thought of driving by herself also made her feel anxious and stressed. She was reluctant to ask her doctor when she could resume driving, fearful that his answer would verify her worst fear: a permanent lifestyle of severely limited freedom and mobility.

Because stress is subject to individual interpretation and experience, concrete lists of what is and isn't stressful don't apply. A limitation that was stressful to Julie, for example, might be a source of relief for another heart patient.

The Myths about Stress

What stress is and how it works to our benefit or harm is not yet clear. Although the consequences of stress levels are largely unknown, many cardiac recovery decisions are based on myths about the efficacy of reducing stress. But some experts agree that stress can be both beneficial and harmful.

Dr. Hans Selye's definitive book, *The Stress of Life,* considers the question of whether stress factors in the environment actually produce harmful effects. His findings reinforce the idea that stress is a necessary part of a person's life.[5]

> The notion that a stress-free life is a more meaningful or qualitatively better life is a myth.

Eliminating stress from anyone's life is impossible. Creating and living in a controlled environment, totally devoid of stimulus or conflict, makes for boredom and a meaningless existence. A certain amount of stress is necessary to remain vital. "Life without stress is death," Dr. Selye contends.

Michael, a minister of a large congregation for twenty-five years, had a heart attack. On the advice of his physician, he retired from his beloved calling because the work was too stressful. He became increasingly depressed and apathetic, wandering around at home like a captain without a ship. Between income from Nancy's work as a medical technician and a pension Michael received from their church's national office, they were able to make ends meet. But financial security didn't resolve the stress of the loss Michael had sustained: the loss of meaningful work and the ability to make a contribution to his community.

Who can say which was more stressful: to practice ministry, feeling needed and connected but heavily stressed by the demanding nature of the work, or to be a depressed pensioner with minimal life stress? What were the consequences of reversing roles, with Nancy becoming the major breadwinner and Michael being stripped of his life's calling?

Live and Learn: Managing Stress

Michael and Nancy's story clearly illustrates the complexity of stress. Each unique situation must be addressed if good decisions involving emotional stress and its effects are going to be made. It also demonstrates how important it is to be an active participant in concert with healthcare professionals you trust. Lifestyle decisions have lasting effects on you and your mate.[6]

Physical stress differs from emotional stress in that it can be measured. A "stress test" can determine a safe level of physical activity for the patient (and heartmate, if necessary), and should be heeded as a guide for physical exertion. Heartmate and partner can set physical limitations. When a patient's job is physical in nature, stress test results may define necessary reductions in work activity. Stress tests also serve medical diagnoses and provide progress reports for recovering patients.

The condition of your marriage or relationship may add physical and emotional stress to your lives. Heart disease demands much, physically and emotionally, from patient and heartmate. Relationships can be complex on the best of days. In a crisis, each of you is more likely to be impatient and intolerant. Fear, anxiety, and physical and emotional exertion can exacerbate stress and irritability, so that things you used to accept and ignore suddenly are a big deal.

> Don't judge the quality of your relationship in the midst of crisis and change.

Fortunately for many, a love relationship is generally a supportive system and a haven. Even if your relationship is a major source of stress at the moment, keep in mind that the familiarity and continuity it provides are important anchors during what would otherwise be a chaotic period. Your relationship wasn't perfect before; why should all the problems magically disappear now?

> This is a time to be especially gentle and under-
> standing with each other. Talk to each other about
> your stress and what you need to manage it.

Reaffirm the support in your relationship. Take time out from each other when things get heated. Seek the support of friends, family, or professionals if needed. Strive to remember that as you become more comfortable with your situation, your stress levels will diminish and your love and understanding are likely to strengthen.

From Caring to Caretaking

A great deal of your time and energy is devoted to looking after the needs of your recovering mate. One reason that you've taken on so much responsibility is because you care. But that's not the only reason. You may also do "caretaking" habitually. Just as there is a distinction between right responsibility and overresponsibility, caring and caretaking are two different things.

Caring is a balance of concern and action, where both the giver and receiver maintain their dignity and power. True caring comes from the heart, and both people feel loved and cared for whether they are giving or receiving.

Caretaking, on the other hand, defines an unequal relationship in which one partner may feel strong, the other weak. Caretakers may unwittingly use the patients' needs against them. When that happens, the patient usually feels obligated, resentful, and helpless. In her book *Helping Yourself Help Others: A Book for Caregivers*, Rosalynn Carter suggests that caregivers can feel powerless, too.

When caregivers perceive themselves as being alone and in "second place" with no one to talk to or help out, they often feel trapped— literally imprisoned in their own households. These feelings can lead to intense anger and depression.

Helplessness and fear are the primary motivating feelings behind caretaking behavior. These feelings are an assault on your sense of power. When you see your spouse vulnerable or in pain, you feel help- less and fearful. You wish that you could do something to fix it. You may also feel fearful about abandonment, loss. You can't change the reality of your mate's heart disease, so you attempt to manage your own feelings of fear and helplessness by caretaking. Most of the time heartmates don't even realize that they are disregarding how their mates feel as a result of their caretaking actions.

Consider the heartmate whose partner refused to quit smoking. Everyone knows that smoking is high on the list of risk factors for heart disease. Each cigarette her partner smoked added to her sense of powerlessness and her growing fear of losing her mate. She felt the pain, sadness, and fear that goes with watching a spouse self-destruct. She nagged, cajoled, begged, blamed, and got angry to try to get him to quit. Nothing worked.

> Caretaking—yes, even nagging and cajoling are forms of caretaking—provides an illusion of con- trol, but in the long run, it's a losing game.

The fact is that the caretaking heartmate is just as powerless over her mate's thoughts, feelings, and behavior as she is over heart disease or the weather. Her attempts to control the uncontrollable inevitably lead to frustration, anxiety, resentment, disempowerment, and low self-esteem.

Women in our culture learn early to be caretakers. Beginning at a young age, girls are rewarded for being sensitive to other people's feel- ings; by adulthood they may be unable to recognize their own. When asked, many adult women find it impossible to know or say what they need. They have suppressed or denied their needs in deference to those of others. Caretaking requires the caretaker to abandon herself for another person.

As much as women today value independence and express resentment about being caretakers, we tend to fall back to this familiar role when we are in crisis, especially if this behavior was ingrained in our youth. Being a caretaker provides the illusion of control, masks helplessness, and keeps us from getting our own needs met.

> Your self-image contributes to your tendency to be a caretaker.

The stereotype of the "good woman" or the "little woman" is a portrait of a gentle, sweet, even-tempered, and, inherently, long-suffering woman. Many women have been conditioned to strive for this ideal, and they struggle to maintain such a picture of themselves, even during a crisis. (If you have low self-esteem, you may be more prone to caretaking as an attempt to boost your sense of self-worth.)

Everything is at risk, and the tools the "good woman" has at hand are sweetness and a willingness to suffer for her man. (The "good man," similarly, may strive to be rescuer and hero, and neglect his own needs in a similar situation.) She doesn't or won't recognize her own feelings. She doesn't know she has needs. She doesn't know that *recovery from her crisis demands that she take care of herself.* She has not been granted permission to express her resentment about having to care for a mate who may not be caring for himself. Or worse, she may be caring for a mate who is only caring about himself.

> Recovery from crisis demands that you take care of yourself.

When the "good woman" maintains the caretaker role, she betrays the very foundation of caring for a sweetness that has soured. This is because caretaking guarantees a loss of mutual respect and admiration. If you take care of your mate's thoughts, feelings, behaviors—his life—he will likely become dependent on you, and sooner or later you both will become resentful.

Popular wisdom encourages caretaking. A commonly held premise is that the heart patient's recovery is in the hands of his spouse. It isn't! You may feel personally responsible for your mate's health, recovery, and even his life. But you're not. Recognize this feeling as a symptom of your caretaking. *You didn't cause his heart disease, and you can't cure it.* You can, however, be a source of support, balancing your assistance, encouragement, and love with caring for yourself.

Loving Detachment

Expressing your caring, rather than becoming a caretaker, is a delicate balance. It requires you to stay in touch with your caring for both your mate and yourself and to respect your partner's right to choose how he lives *his life.* Remember, no one can "make" another person change. You are rightly powerless over your partner.

Practicing loving detachment is difficult; it is especially difficult when you see your partner refusing to make heart-healthy lifestyle choices—contrary to your wishes. Your efforts to control will be activated by your fears. Sometimes, for example, heartmates turn to blame or shame in an effort to coerce their mates to quit smoking, eat carefully, take medications religiously, exercise regularly, and eliminate unnecessary stress.

When you begin to blame and shame, it's probably time to detach. You are helpless to do anything that can make your spouse take his illness seriously. The greater your fear, for example, the more the patient pushes himself, ignoring prescribed physical limitations. Many patients are admitted "workaholics" and may strongly resist changing or limiting their careers in response to their heart condition. Others' resistance may be related to denial or resignation.

Your internal need to caretake will probably be in direct proportion to your mate's resistance. The more he pushes himself, the more you nag him to slow down. If he makes a joke about eating steak, you counter with a lecture on the evils of cholesterol. You interpret anything less than perfection (the instant reversal of decades-long habit) as denial or irresponsibility. If his attitude reflects a lack of concern for his condition, you will feel a need to redouble your efforts, and you will exhaust yourself on his behalf. This is a time to state your concerns and detach. You can really only take care of yourself.

Beyond behaviors, you may find yourself caretaking your mate's feelings, too. Male heart patients, for example, traditionally ignore and deny their feelings. They may mask their insecurity, fear, and sadness with bravado and machismo. You may consciously or unconsciously take on and express your partner's unexpressed feelings. At one time or another, you've probably said or felt, "I'm worrying for both of us."

> There's danger to you both in assuming your mate's feelings. You can't carry the burden without a cost to yourself.

Consequences include your sense of failure, depression, even despair. Your genuine concern and desire to emotionally protect your mate will ultimately backfire, with a negative result for him, too. If your mate doesn't have to deal with his own feelings, he can't recover from the emotional dimension of his cardiac crisis.

> Caring about your mate doesn't mean doing everything for him, especially at the expense of your own needs. This is called caretaking and self-abandonment.

You can care and also lovingly detach. Ultimately, it is not your responsibility to make your spouse recover. You can help. You can be supportive.[7] You can care. But you do not have the power to save his life. No person has that power over another. Genuine caring involves letting go and encouraging your mate's independence.

Making the Shift from Caretaker to Partner

Clearly, there are negative consequences for acting in an overresponsible way, for caretaking. A relationship of caretaker and victim/ patient fosters dependency, resentment, and loss of self, all of which slow the physical and emotional recovery of your mate—and you.

Many years ago the treatment for a heart attack was weeks of bed rest, sometimes months. Current information, however, establishes that lying in bed weakens rather than strengthens patients. Muscles that aren't used tend to atrophy. The old mode of treatment also tended to encourage dependency and caretaking.

Trying to limit your spouse's physical activity by doing everything for him directly opposes modern medical wisdom. Today, cardiac patients are encouraged to begin walking soon after a heart attack or after surgery. Cardiac rehabilitation programs are now based on a carefully modulated regimen of activity interspersed with rest. Caretaking simply isn't indicated.

Encouraging your mate's dependence can be psychologically and emotionally damaging for him (and you). Patients struggle with the challenge of holding on to their self-respect. Perception of self-worth can be negatively affected by the stigma associated with heart disease. Rebuilding a healthy self-image happens gradually, as your mate successfully handles more and more while integrating realistic limitations.

Building a positive, healthy self-image and attitude takes motivation and confidence. If you persist in taking over for your mate, he may start to wonder if his condition is more serious than he's been told. Doing things for him that he's capable of doing for himself makes him feel handicapped and inadequate. In response to all the "help" he received from his spouse, one patient reported, "It's as if having a heart attack curdled my brain." After a while, an individual who sees himself as an invalid will begin to believe that he is truly in-valid. No cardiac spouse wants to contribute to such a negative attitude.

When you take too much responsibility for your mate, you also hamper your own recovery. If you're continually taking care of him, you are probably not taking care of yourself. How can you be present for your mate, be a partner in recovery, if you're not healthy yourself?

Trapped in overresponsibility and caretaking, neither of you is meeting your recovery needs. Both of you may be strained by a relationship that needs caring, not caretaking, right responsibility, not overresponsibility. When stress levels in the relationship escalate, both of you feel smothered; neither feels recognized, supported, or affirmed.

> Follow the Heartmates Five-Step Plan for Right Responsibility to orient yourself and strengthen your relationship.

If you feel that you're doing well detaching and sharing and balancing responsibilities, congratulate yourself! If not, you can start practicing these new recovery behaviors today. Regardless of where you are with these behaviors, the following five steps are a good guide for practicing right responsibility.

HEARTMATES®
FIVE-STEP PLAN FOR RIGHT RESPONSIBILITY

Step 1: Accept your powerlessness. Accepting powerlessness over others, events, and circumstances is easier said than done, but it is the critical first step in establishing right responsibility. Until you can accept that caretaking and controlling are running your life, you will be shortsighted, your perceptions distorted. Continuous attempts at managing the unmanageable lead you down a road of frustration and heartache.

Step 2: Assess your situation realistically. You know more about your situation than any expert or outsider. Strive to be realistic about which responsibilities are exigent and which you can let go. Don't downplay or overdramatize your situation.

Step 3: Look honestly at your own behavior. Without blame or self-deprecation, observe your behaviors in the recovery process and evaluate the positive and negative consequences of those behaviors to you, to your mate, and to your relationship. Check your motives. Are your behaviors governed by fear, obligation, and a need to control, or are they based on caring, sharing, loving, giving, and receiving.

Step 4: Differentiate between right responsibility and overresponsibility, caring and caretaking. Use the results from step 3 to guide you in determining where your thinking and behavior might be showing signs of overresponsibility and caretaking. You may want to discuss steps 3 and 4 with your spouse or a trusted confidante to help you determine the difference.

Step 5: Make changes. The direction of change should be relative to where you are in recovery. As time passes and you move farther away from the acute period of physical care, begin to shift your attention from your mate's health to your own. Your recovery frees you and your mate to take on right responsibility and caring, reestablishing or reaffirming your individual sense of self-worth and well-being. It will also open you both to mutual respect and true intimacy.

> Gradually wean yourself from the responsibility of being available for any and every demand.

As the weeks and months go by, return to other aspects and activities of your life. At first the change may be small: leaving the house for a short time to do some shopping or meeting a friend for lunch. The next separate excursion may be a concert or community meeting. It may be advisable to work up to a bigger separation, such as taking a day trip to a spa, attending a weekend retreat, or visiting one of your grown children for a few days.

These steps are part of *your* recovery process. They take time, effort, commitment, and courage. No change comes easily. Lifelong habits conditioned by early training and cultural acceptance are very difficult to change.

Don't underestimate the healing power of sharing these ideas with other heartmates. You don't have to be alone with all the change you are experiencing. You can encourage each other when the situation is difficult and your progress seems slow. Find someone you trust to cheer you on. Celebrate as you take steps to further your personal recovery.

Chapter 5 Notes

1. Bishop Clarkson Hospital in Omaha, Nebraska, uses beepers for heartmates to support them during hospital stays—their cardiac spouses are fortunate indeed.
2. Stanton Peele and Archie Brodsky, *Love and Addiction* (New York: New American Library, 1975), 6.
3. In *Mainstay: For the Well Spouse of the Chronically Ill*, Maggie Strong gives the well spouse permission to feel bad about, resent, even hate the unchosen burden of responsibility when a partner becomes chronically ill—all without guilt.
4. Robert Eliot, MD, *Stress and the Major Cardiovascular Disorders* (Mt. Kisco, N.Y.: Futura Publishing, 1979), 14.
5. Hans Selye, MD, *The Stress of Life* (New York: McGraw Hill, 1956), 299. See appendix D in this book for an essay on stress written by massage therapist and health educator, Pamela R. Borgmann, BA, RN, MTh.
6. I have been fortunate to have the opportunity to learn from William J. Doherty, PhD, coauthor of *Families and Health* and *Medical Family Therapy*, in a variety of professional settings. His groundbreaking work envisions collaborative healthcare systems staffed by professionals who respect and acknowledge the needs and difficulties of spouses who have assumed the role of caregiver in families organized around a chronic illness. His ethical stance emphasizes factoring in everyone's need to achieve the goals of agency (autonomy) and communion (interpersonal connection) with the family.
7. Regarding the efficacy of support and optimism, quoting [italics mine] from a 1998 German study, "Predicting Cardiac Patients' Quality of Life from the Characteristics of Their Spouses" (Freie Universität Berlin): *"Optimistic partners* who see themselves as *active agents of their own life can be resourceful support persons* who help to improve a patient's readjustment after his or her cardiac surgery." (See also chapter 4 about the importance of optimism.)

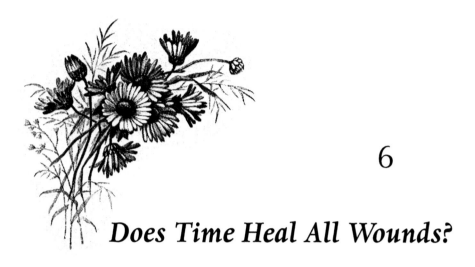

6

Does Time Heal All Wounds?

M*y identity permanently changed when I became a heartmate. I no longer believed that I had complete control over my life and my destiny. There was nothing I could do to alter the fact that my husband had heart disease. I came to accept that I live in an imperfect world in which unexpected change, change beyond my control, can occur at any moment.*

I lost my innocence. My belief in my own immortality and that of those I loved was gone. In one shocking moment, my naiveté vanished. In its place were fear of loss, abandonment, and the unknown. My husband's brushes with death made me realize that our time on earth is limited, that we will not live forever.

My wounds were so deep, I hurt to my very core. My beliefs and dreams of a secure future were gone. I felt afraid to live, to love. I resented life for its unpredictability. I yearned to feel secure and alive again, to have my trust in life restored.

Time did diminish my pain, and I came to see the gift in the experience. I came to see the bounds of my control. I learned to live despite the reality of uncertainty. I saw that I had been squandering time, as if I had eternity tucked in my back pocket. I learned to set my priorities more thoughtfully.

The pain of heart disease is pervasive and enduring, like the disease itself. The original trauma passes, but it leaves permanent change. It wounds and scars your body, mind, and spirit.

Fortunately, time is on your side. Your mate has survived and so have you. As the weeks and months pass, you find reassurance that life goes on. Time has taught you a number of things. You're no longer afraid to leave your mate at home, and you're less involved with his physical symptoms. You've come through the crisis with increased strength, resilience, and adaptability.

But your journey isn't over. Everything has changed, and even time can't make things "normal" again. You can't cancel what has happened.

Our cultural conditioning perpetuates the myth that if you're good and do everything right, your pain will vanish and you'll live happily ever after. But you're not living a fairy tale; this is life, your life. There is no magic that can make the recent past disappear. There are no pills or time machines to transport you back to an earlier time of innocence. The cardiac spouse faces countless disappointments, including a suddenly altered future and broken dreams.[1] Your spouse's heart disease has affected your lifestyle, your financial security, your marital relationship, your most deeply held beliefs, your very identity.

You probably now question everything: your values, ideas, and convictions, even who you are. If you always believed that your mate is stronger than you, his physical weakness and vulnerability caused by heart disease threaten this belief. If you measured your intimacy by the degree of passion in your sexual relationship, new limitations invite a reevaluation of your perceptions.

Firmly held ideas, such as "Nothing bad can happen if you believe in God or a higher power" or "These things happen to other people," are now meaningless. You may feel confused and betrayed. The crisis shattered your security and demolished your precious dreams. Something is very, very wrong. You have arrived at that universal and dramatic realization that *nothing will ever be the same.*

Confronting permanent change can be devastating. Heart disease exacts its costs: limited activity, lost security, and painful adjustments in your personal relationships. Your feelings of sadness and anger are valid, whether they are in reaction to something small, like giving up your favorite foods, or more profound, like relinquishing long-term plans for the future.

Becoming a heartmate forces removal of your rose-colored glasses. Your mate's heart disease has brought you face to face with your own personal reality, including the wounds you carry from your losses. You've lost things you deeply valued: in your work, recreational, private, and family life; in your routine and lifestyle; and in your heart of hearts, where your long-held dreams, values, and priorities reside.

Why, in this era of medical miracles, is there no cure for heart disease? Why is heart disease irreversible and permanent? Why do you and your partner have to cope with heart disease? Answers are not apparent. But asking "why?" and "why me?" point to a broken value system. These legitimate questions may have no answers, but they signal that your process of mourning and healing has begun.

Change demands that we grieve, but *grieving is not negative*. You must grieve to fully heal. Grief is healing. Just as there is no end without a beginning, there is no loss without the possibility of gain. In the cardiac crisis, there is a positive path to traverse and a chance for personal healing and growth.

Wisdom of the ages includes the Tao definition of crisis as "opportunity" and Hippocrates' perception that "healing is a matter of time, but it is sometimes also a matter of opportunity."[2] *Carpe diem*. In our time, no one has advocated better for hope, healing, and humor than Norman Cousins, who claimed, "Healing is possible, even when curing is not."[3] Grief is the human process that makes acceptance and healing possible.

Grief and Loss

Human life includes loss and death. Perhaps one of the most difficult things we face is learning how to absorb and survive loss—how to "let go." Some losses are easier to accept than others.

Grief, commonly understood to be limited to the emotional process following a death, is, in fact, part of all change. Every change we experience has two elements, loss and potential gain. To accept and adapt to the losses accompanying heart disease, as well as see and accept potential gains, you need to identify and grieve your losses.

The cardiac crisis includes many and diverse losses.[4] Having dealt with one pain, it can be a surprise and disappointment to find that down the road there is yet another to confront. For most heartmates, loss of the familiar and, perhaps, comfortable life they had before the cardiac crisis is one of the most difficult. You will probably wish for your old life. Longing for the past is a normal and natural part of grief. Remembering and honoring what was an important component of grieving your losses. This is mourning.

The custom of mourning is as old as life itself. Our cultural past is rich with wisdom. The original Sanskrit definition of mourning means "remembering." In Greek, mourning means "caring." Our current understanding of mourning includes both components. Centuries ago, the rabbis of Judea codified rituals of mourning. The first year after a loss was divided into smaller parts: the first week, the first month, and the first eleven months. Observances and rituals for each period were defined, giving families permission to mourn and providing a guide for "working through" grief.

And our modern world is rich with wisdom about mourning, too. "For mourning is the constant reawakening that things are now different."[5] The Yakima Indian Nation gives us: "Mourning makes peace with change."[6] Explaining her belief that grieving is among the most fundamental of life skills, Rachel Naomi Remen, MD, says, "If it were up to me, [grieving] would be taught in kindergarten, right up there with taking turns and sharing."[7]

Mourning is painful emotional and spiritual work; yet, mourning is how we experience and express our grief, heal the pain. As you mourn, you will probably ache over feeling vulnerable and helpless. There will be the mental pain of not understanding. Your intellectual mind needs to understand the loss, to find acceptance and establish meaning in what seems so pointless. And finally, there is the pain that is hunger for significance, the yearning to transform tragedy into something good.

Elisabeth Kübler-Ross, whose monumental work lifted the cultural taboo of silence about loss and death, suggested stages through which mourners pass: denial, anger or resentment, bargaining, sadness or depression, acceptance. People don't always experience the stages in order; some move back and forth from stage to stage. Others experience several stages simultaneously. Even mourners who have reached the stage of acceptance may continue at times to wrestle with pain and fears and yearn for the past. Kübler-Ross' courageous writing legitimized the grieving process for all of us.

> *Mourning can go on for years and years. It doesn't end after a year; that's a false fantasy. It usually ends when people realize that they can live again, that they can concentrate their energies on their lives as a whole, and not on their hurt, and guilt, and pain.*[8]

Although professional literature has established the validity and therapeutic value of grief, we are still under social pressure to keep our mourning responses brief. We are a people journeying in the fast lane, intolerant of and impatient with anything that is slower than jet speed or cannot be neatly resolved within the span of a television drama. Our culture adds to our burden and undermines our self-esteem by ignoring and avoiding the individual's normal need to grieve losses.

> Despite pressure to "hurry up and get on with life," allow yourself all the time and attention you need to grieve and mourn.

The pace of each person's experience of grieving is unique. You are at your most vulnerable, and you need to proceed through grief in your own way, even when our culture fails to give you a model, a guide, or unqualified support. You have a right to your grief.

> *Illness, and perhaps only illness, gives us permission to slow down. . . . Illness restores the sense of proportion that is lost when we take life for granted. . . . Among the basic rights that should belong to every human is that of experiencing what is happening to oneself. . . . To grieve well is to value what you have lost. When you value even the feeling of loss, you value life itself, and you begin to live again.*[9]

The cardiac spouse's losses are real and important. In *All Our Losses/All Our Griefs*, Kenneth R. Mitchell and Herbert Anderson describe symbolic, intrapsychic losses as "the experience of losing an emotionally important image of oneself, losing the possibilities of 'what might have been,' abandonment of plans for a particular future, and the dying of a dream."[10]

You must grieve these losses in order to live fully in the present and plan for the future. If you don't permit yourself to grieve, you may get psychologically stuck. Grief may reduce your ability to cope with and adapt to the reality of heart disease. It may also result in physical symptoms such as chronic headaches, tension, and illness. (Grieving people are more susceptible to physical ailments and illnesses for up to two years after a crisis. Those who fail to grieve, however, have an increased susceptibility to illness.)

In resisting your grief, you deny yourself the good seeds born of grieving, seeds vital for planting a new crop of realistic dreams for the garden of your future. Trust yourself and the grief process. Your efforts will bear fruit.

> *The reward of mourning is realized as the survivor sheds her [old] . . . identity and dares to hope for new relationships. . . . The restorative power of mourning and the extraordinary human capacity for renewal after even the most profound loss is evident. . . .*[11]

In grieving, you will move from what was to what is, from who you *were* to who you *are*—stronger, wiser, and with a greater capacity to live and love.

The Healing Process

If your wounds were obvious, involving scars or other survival badges, friends and family would better understand your need to take the time to heal. But *your wounds are not so visible.* Judging by your appearance, many people probably assume that you are healthy and whole. And in some ways, you are, but you are still grieving, performing the difficult and painful work of coming to accept the permanent changes heart disease has brought you.

Healing is a highly individual process. Each person has distinct needs and timing. Treat yourself kindly. Don't pressure yourself to rush through this. Don't push yourself faster than you can go, and don't let others, uncomfortable or impatient with your pace, pressure you into activities or decisions for which you're not yet ready.

Time is central to the healing process, but time alone is *not* enough. To cleanse and treat your wounds, confront your losses. Deny, blame, bargain, rage, despair—mourn.

> Tell your story. Talk about your circumstances and struggles.

The gift of acceptance will allow you to make peace with what has happened, with your and your spouse's imperfection and vulnerability, and with the change that is inherent in living. It will allow you to reconnect to yourself (your new identity in the present, with your memories and your realistic hopes for the future intact), your mate, and your life.

When you are recovering from a loss, such as the vicarious trauma of a loved one's heart disease, the process of grief and healing is essentially the same as with grieving a death. Here are some guidelines that may assist you in your grief process:

1. Recognize and name your wounds.
2. Face reality.
3. Release your feelings.
4. Update your images.
5. Forgive.

Recognizing and Naming Your Wounds

It's natural to try to avoid pain. One way is to ignore what's happened. That may be easy for you to do if your mate has had a full physical recovery. He may look healthier than he has in years. Often, recovered bypass patients have ruddy complexions and report that they're feeling great. But behind the complexion and assurances, painful feelings remain. You can imagine your partner's feelings when you read this heart patient's journal, written after her bypass surgery:

> *My primary concerns just days after bypass surgery were hardly about whether a man would still find me attractive or whether my children would be embarrassed by me. I was apprehensive about my chances for recovery, the effects of heart disease on my energy, my work, my priorities, my life.*
>
> *I faced so many unanswerable questions. Was I going to survive? What was lost to me now? Would I ever again experience the sense of control over my life that I had taken so for granted before? Would my family and friends still love the changed me?*
>
> *It became more and more difficult to examine or question when those around me kept saying, "You look great; you were really lucky!" I didn't feel great or lucky. I felt traumatized, scared, vulnerable, outraged, confused, and so sad. I needed time—time I wasn't all that sure I had. I didn't know what my physical or emotional or mental losses would be. I did know that I would never again be the woman I'd been before surgery. I was changed forever. But who was I?*

Just as this patient felt devalued and unseen by those who urged her to look on the bright side, so, too, do painful feelings remain for heartmates. Glossing over the totality of change and the prospect of the unknown is an attempt to avoid mourning by trivializing it. This is denial. You may hear others suggest to you, or you may even tell yourself, that this is no big deal. You might follow up the thought with an attempt to live your life exactly as it was before heart disease. Fearful of being self-pitying, you may ask, "What in the world have I got to complain about?" denying yourself permission to examine very real wounds.

Where you are in your life when heart disease sets in is a critical component determining the scope and depth of your pain. Young cardiac couples, for example, will face the concern and strain of deciding whether or not they should have a family, or even if they should stay together. Not many years later, heart disease may be complicated with child-rearing issues, including concerns about children and adolescents who are struggling with a parent's heart disease. Older couples, having made sacrifices for their family, experience the disappointment of broken dreams for their own future. Heart disease cheats them out of their leisure years, a time they believed would be restful or adventurous.

Trying to deny or otherwise escape pain only sends it underground. Wounds need fresh air to heal. Like an infection that must run its course, incurable with a Band-Aid, your crisis won't disappear even if you feign a cure or pretend that it doesn't exist.

> Feelings exist and persist. They need to be felt, expressed, and released.

Denial obstructs the recovery process and diminishes your freedom and spontaneity, your ability to live fully.

Marilyn, the fifty-one-year-old wife of a cardiac bypass patient, shared an extreme, but not unusual, example of the pitfalls of denial. She proudly described how she avoided her feelings about Robert's surgery. She worked out a plan so she'd never see his scars. The last thing she wanted was to be reminded of the nightmare they'd been through. Marilyn made sure she wasn't in their bedroom when Robert was dressing or undressing. She got into bed only after he had turned out the light, so she wouldn't see his bare chest. If Robert sat by their apartment-house pool in his swimming trunks, Marilyn would find something to do that kept her inside.

This carefully wrought plan required more and more of Marilyn's energy and attention. What began as a solution, a way to treat her pain, ended up a trap. Marilyn's daily life became dictated by her denial. After many months, Marilyn realized how disengaged she was from herself and Robert. With the support of a professional counselor, she got through her denial and began to feel again.

Recognizing your wounds may be difficult because you weren't raised to identify and value your own feelings and needs. You may be so conditioned in the role of caretaker that you honestly don't know that you have been hurt. A successful caretaker puts in twenty-four-hour days, makes every effort to take care of others, combats the inevitable. The caretaker doesn't know how to assess her own feelings, goes, in fact, to great lengths to shut them off. In time, she learns to do so instinctively. She has been given no permission to let down or let go; how she feels is the least of her worries. She's always on duty, perennially cheerful, and indefatigable, even after years of service.

Untrained and unsupported in feeling emotions, the caretaker fears them and what they might mean. What might happen if you move beyond denial and habit to challenge that deep and universal fear of the unknown? Will you survive if you remove the Band-Aids and see your wounds? Will you drown in your tears or find them a comfort and a relief? What proof is there that if you confront your despair—that which is lost, outdated, or gone—there'll be anything to replace it?

Fear of the unknown can be fought only with faith and courage. The reward is wholeness and peace of mind.

> *Courage is the price that life exacts*
> *for granting peace.*
> *The souls that know it not,*
> *know no release from little things.*[12]

Recognizing your wounds does not guarantee positive growth in and of itself. Recognition is the necessary springboard into your grief work.

> With faith that there is something beyond your grief and the courage to act in the face of your fear and pain, you will come to name and mourn your losses.

Facing Reality

In your process of healing, it is important to discern what your losses mean to you. Thinking about what has happened and what it means gives definition to your pain and loss and lays the groundwork for figuring out how you can heal from them, what you need to take care of yourself.

A wound heals well only after its severity and a treatment plan are determined. To fully grasp what you have lost, *review* (re-view) and *relive* your experience—it's an integral part of grieving. (See appendix A, "Self-Help Resources," for the Evening Review, particularly useful because it provides a simple review structure. Reviewing is a mental activity that helps a person to think clearly, see reality, and establish order in the chaos of the crisis.)

One of the best ways to understand your pain is to name it and then talk about it. Seek out friends who can be present for you as you tell your story. Plan outings, such as lunch in the back booth at your favorite restaurant, or a secluded walk by the lake or in the woods, where you can talk undisturbed. You might also consider attending a support group.

> Share your story and listen to the stories of others. They will help you gain perspective, understanding, and healing.

Prepare your story, relying on your memory, your feelings, and the reviewing skills in this book. Strive to determine the scope of your story. Reconstruct your life "before" the cardiac event, during the crisis, and your present circumstances. Include your relationship, your ideals, dreams, and plans. Don't forget your struggles and conflicts.

Then tell your story. Share what life was like before the crisis, what changes were thrust upon you, what your life is like now. As difficult as it may be, include your bodily sensations and your feelings. These details are as important as the facts (sharing them also will give them recognition, voice, and release). And, finally, share what you think it all means to you. As you tell your story, you may realize that you've lost facts and details. Contact the doctor, family members, or anyone who might provide clarity to and validation of your memories.

Your story will change. With each retelling, as missing details are remembered, as your feelings become more apparent, as your understanding becomes more precise, as you find sense and meaning, your story will echo your progress in healing. Gail Sher, Zen practitioner and contemporary writer, affirms this crucial restorative nature of storytelling in her 1999 book, *One Continuous Mistake:*

> *Implicit in every syllable of our uninterrupted inner monologue is testimony to an entire life. Retelling it (like prayer) becomes a way of relinquishing, a way of overcoming.*

Psychologist Shelley Taylor, too, has done extensive research linking recovery with people's ability to tell their stories.[13] Her studies indicate that "tragedy brings forth the need to create meaning—to tell new stories—that can reweave the frayed ends of life into a coherent whole."

> Reviewing and sharing your experience helps you separate the reality of what has happened from your feelings about what happened.

Keep talking. Over a period of time it will become clear to you what you experienced, how you have and are responding, and how your life has changed.

By storytelling, you are constructing the foundation for a new, more realistic image of your experience, your feelings, and yourself. Supportive listeners who are willing to witness your experience and keep it confidential can also serve as a reality check. As you talk, you'll begin to explore important questions, such as the following, that help you face, test, and challenge your reality. They also provide you with greater understanding of what you need to do to take care of yourself:

- How does my spouse's heart condition really affect me?
- What is most important now in my life?

- What's realistic for me to expect of myself now?
- How do I feel about the ways in which our relationship has changed?

Releasing Feelings

Facing reality uncovers your feelings. At this point in your healing process, you will probably begin feeling the sadness, hurt, disappointment, and anger associated with your losses. You may feel overwhelmed or out of control. But the pain of knowing is also cleansing. If you've been unable to cry since all this began, for example, your tears may come now. Imagine them cleansing your wounds and offering relief—a loving gift to yourself.

> If you can, allow yourself to cry with someone you trust and who will support you.

Many heartmates have found sharing their stories with a skilled, empathetic therapist or grief counselor to be helpful. If you are having difficulty forming or sharing your story, consider consulting a professional yourself. Good therapists and grief counselors will support your expression of feelings, help you test reality and take responsibility for your recovery, and eventually assist you in the reconstruction of a reality that makes sense. These professionals can also help you form an action plan for coping with change and stepping fully into *a new life* that includes heart disease.

Our culture traditionally views the expression of feelings as a sign of weakness. Yet, the opposite is true. The release of emotion, through words, tears, gestures, is healing and requires the utmost courage. Only the strong dare to share their true feelings. Your feelings indicate how deeply affected you are by your losses. Shakespeare's advice in *Macbeth* applies to cardiac spouses today: "Give sorrow words; the grief that does not speak whispers the o'er fraught heart and bids it break."[14]

> Writing is a good way to "give sorrow words," to
> acknowledge, explore, and release your feelings.

Writing is another way of telling your story. Consider keeping a journal, and use it to communicate with yourself. Set aside time every day. Sit in a safe and comfortable place. Tune in to your thoughts and feelings, and write in your journal. (Review chapter note 7 on page 104 about the value and rewards of journal writing.)

Anger may be the most difficult emotion for you to acknowledge, and its power may be one of the "surprises" you experience related to your partner's cardiac crisis. Many heartmates deny their anger as a method of coping with it. Some see their anger as a sign of weakness and selfishness. Others don't feel entitled to their anger and try to minimize it or explain it away. Heartmates also feel ashamed of their anger. You may argue, for example, that you weren't widowed by heart disease, so you have no right to be angry. One cardiac spouse told me that anger was a sin.

Acknowledging, feeling, and releasing your anger is hard but necessary work. Doing so may feel like the first fatal step on the road to total disintegration, loss of control. It isn't. Anger is a normal human response to hurt and loss. You can't reach acceptance without dealing with your anger. Letting go of your anger requires that you stop holding on to it, protecting it, hiding it from yourself and others. The true control of your anger lies in acknowledging, accepting, and feeling it.

When you feel bad for being angry, even acknowledging it can prompt a sense of unworthiness and low self-esteem. (When you feel bad about your anger, you abandon yourself, rejecting a normal and healthy part of your humanity.)

> Remember, anger is only a feeling. It is not a
> measure of your worth and being.

You can't work through your anger unless you first acknowledge that you have it. Only your behavior is truly open to judgment.

You're probably angry about many things. It's conceivable that you feel angry and hurt that your mate has withdrawn since the cardiac crisis. Perhaps you feel sorely in need of care and affection, emotionally deprived. Or maybe you're furious that your spouse has not appreciated your extra effort on his behalf over these months. The cardiac experience presents a multitude of things to feel angry about.

One of the most common signs of unexpressed anger is blaming. You may blame the doctor, the professional staff, the entire hospital system for what's happened to your spouse, to you, and for how you're feeling. You may be angry at your spouse, blaming him for having heart disease, for smoking, for being a "type A," or even for his genetic predisposition for heart disease.

Regardless of the nature and strength of your faith, you might find yourself angry at God or your higher power. Harvey, who had been very religious, felt as though God had turned his back on him. Caroline described how unfair it was for God to abandon her after she had "been good" all her life. Yet another heartmate believed that God was punishing her with the heart disease. It is common and natural for heartmates to be angry with their higher power about their circumstances. It's just as common for them to instinctively hide this anger.

Your health and recovery depend on your acknowledging, feeling, expressing, and releasing your feelings, including your anger. Holding on to anger will isolate you and add to the emotional distance between you, others, and God. If you don't feel and release your anger, it doesn't go away. Like other feelings, it waits to be felt and expressed, often coming out sideways. Stockpiling anger builds resentment and bitterness and creates barriers, cutting you off from the understanding and support of others.

If you risk expressing your feelings to your spouse, you'll probably be amazed at how your perceptions differ. But even if you disagree, you still will have acknowledged and named your anger. It isn't about being fair, accurate, or unselfish. Your anger is based on your perception of your experience.

The same is true of God or your higher power. We can learn to live our faiths, trusting that our relationship with God will not be diminished if we express our feelings, even anger. We can learn that we needn't keep our anger hidden inside. We abandon God and ourselves by withholding our anger. Expressing it, we discover our humanity and that a higher power is present in our lives.

Learning to acknowledge, feel, and release feelings doesn't happen in a day or a week; the process occurs over time, often in small measures. You may, for example, instinctively hesitate to release feelings, certain that doing so will be overpowering. But that is rarely the case. Your psyche, naturally healing itself, will determine a pace that is right and safe for you.

For a while, I went along acting as if everything was okay. I felt numb as I went through the motions of my everyday routine. I forced myself to stay calm, managing the household, the kids, and myself as steadily as I could. Protected by my robot-like efficiency, I told myself I was perfectly capable of handling what had happened.

I had been cautioned that my husband needed rest and no stress in order to heal. How could I tell him that I was afraid he would be disabled or die? How could I tell him I was afraid he'd never work again, that I was frozen with anxiety about money for our family's future? How could I tell him that I was infuriated at him for not taking better care of his body and for causing me all this distress?

How could I tell him that my trust was eroded, now that he'd proved he was not immortal and invincible? How could I tell him how scared I was that he would keel over and die if he missed or was late taking his pills? How could I tell him that I was waking in the middle of the night to listen for his breath, scared he was laying dead beside me? How could I tell him that I was afraid to leave the house, sure that his life was my responsibility, and that I hated it?

Of course, I didn't say these things, at least not aloud, to him or to anyone. Ashamed of my feelings, I kept them hidden deep inside, and I became progressively more isolated and alone. Instead of expressing my fear, I concentrated on my competence. I repaired the back fence with a hammer and nails. I busily painted our bedroom and wallpapered our bathroom. I never considered how he felt, lying in bed recovering, as I frantically painted us into separate corners.

Life became a series of mechanical actions without meaning. Like a coronary artery slowly closing down, the life and love between us got so sluggish it was barely enough to keep our relationship alive.

It was many months later that the incongruity of my behavior hit me. Here I was, acting as if I didn't need him, when there was no one in the world I treasured more. I was terrified of losing him and yet I was pushing him away. Instead of drawing near, I had constructed a wall of bravado between us, trying desperately to prove that I could live without him. After feeling so betrayed, I was determined never to be that vulnerable again. I had decided that if there was a chance of his abandoning me, I would leave first, if not physically, then emotionally. I abandoned him—and myself.

A wave of shame raced through me as I realized what I had done. How could I be so selfish? He was sick and needed me, and I was concerned only with protecting myself. Like a waterfall, tears began to stream down my face. They washed away my shame, and I forgave myself. Feeling released, I made a new and conscious vow to share my love and vulnerability—to be his heartmate.

Acknowledging "what is" gives you the raw material to make a new beginning. With acceptance, you can see how the crisis has affected you. Ventilated sorrow and anger melt away and new compassion toward yourself and your mate emerges. You can't change what has already happened, neither can you turn back time, but once you've faced reality, grieved, and cleansed your wounds, you can move ahead.

The Power of Images

Trust is based on a series of experiences that provide a reliable image of reality. Whether you're aware of it or not, you probably trust in the security of your lifestyle, a stable relationship with your mate, and your expectations of the future. As each day dawns and everything you take for granted in your life continues to be there, your images are supported and reinforced. Until something happens to threaten your images, you continue to place your trust in the world-view you've created.

All heartmates share a loss of trust as our images shatter with the unexpected shock of heart disease. We need to repair our images to complete the process of healing. In the adult world, images are rarely discussed or taken seriously. Images are considered to be the product of children's imaginations, the senility of the aged, or the delusions of the mentally ill.

Imagery combines our mental and emotional perceptions of events. Beyond conscious awareness, our minds and emotions interpret and define reality.

> Our images form the basis of our worldview and are the foundation of our actions. We believe the world is the way we "see it." We respond to our images as if they are reality.

If your image of a hospital is a place with a competent and caring staff, you will feel satisfied with the quality of care your spouse receives. If your image of a hospital is a place of helplessness and isolation, that may give rise to a very different interpretation: that it's an impersonal, untrustworthy place. The truth is probably somewhere in between, but *your image is your reality.*

The power of imagery and of the mind-matter connection are not well understood, but even the superstitious are familiar with the concept of a self-fulfilling prophecy. It's the idea that what we imagine eventually comes to pass. Though the following examples illustrate the power of images in the lives of cardiac patients, that power is not limited to them. It is available to everyone.

A patient overheard staff describing him as "the man with the galloping heart." This is a severe and debilitating condition, yet this patient continued to thrive. Some years later he explained to his doctor that he attributed his amazing recovery to the fact that he had a galloping heart, which he believed meant a robust and rugged heart that would not fail him.

Norman Cousins, author, healer, and heart patient, described seeing medics from an ambulance rush to the aid of a man who had suddenly collapsed as he walked a golf course. The medical personnel were monitoring his blood pressure and pulse. Cousins read the monitor, but seeing that the man looked really scared, he put his hand on the patient's shoulder and told him that he had a very strong heart and was going to make it. Within a minute's time the monitor's dangerously high reading had returned to almost normal.[15]

There is research indicating that when patients make the effort to construct and then believe positive images, visualizing chemicals or rays destroying all the cancer cells in the body, for example, they may actually live longer than patients whose imagery is negative.[16] Statistics on programs using positive imagery to treat or reverse heart disease, though limited, are promising. Cardiac patients who believe they can promote their good health participate in their recovery in positive ways (e.g., committing to food plans and exercise programs) and tend to experience an improved quality of life.

The Influence of Personal Images

If imagery has the power to affect our physical conditions, it seems likely that it would affect our psychological and spiritual health as well. Penny, age thirty-two, sat weeping on a park bench as she watched her twin toddlers playing happily on the swings. She cried, believing she had lost the dream of what she called a "normal" family. She grieved because her family would not have a carefree life now that her husband had heart disease. Her children would no longer be innocent offspring of perfectly healthy parents.

In Penny's mind, serious illness precluded an ideal family. Her ability to cry and her willingness to discuss her lost image were encouraging signs of recovery. Expressing her frustration and disappointment, she began to redefine what normal might mean, and to rebuild her image of her family's future.

When we hold our images up to the mirror of reality, we see a distorted reflection. The pain we experience often depends on how big a gap looms between what's real and what we wish were true. The door of opportunity, the positive side of a crisis, begins to open when we challenge our unexamined images and face what's real.

My husband's heart attack changed my image of who he is. I had never given any thought to his mortality. In the life-threatening crisis that brought him to a bed in the coronary care unit, I saw what I hadn't noticed or thought about until then. He is mortal. This means that he will die. Maybe not now, but he won't live forever.

That thought came as a great surprise! I knew that I would die. I'd realized that when my mother died years earlier. But I had never transferred that awareness to the image I held of my husband. My image of him was that he was invincible. Not only was he physically strong and active, his energy for life seemed so unfaltering.

If I thought far enough into the future, to our eighties or nineties, I could imagine us aged and then dying. This image made sense and was acceptable to me. But the day my image was shattered, I was only forty-three.

He was my first love, my high school sweetheart. My image of him then was of a handsome, blue-eyed blond with an athlete's body, a scholar's mind, an intensity for life, and a powerful moral drive. Had I never looked at him again? Why hadn't I seen the changes time had wrought?

The man I saw looking out at me from the tubes, wires, and machinery in the cardiac care unit that night was a half-bald, gray-faced, middle-aged man. Where had my adolescent hero gone? Who was this sick and aging man, his blue eyes flecked with fear and disbelief? Was I married to my father, my grandfather?

Why had I never noticed time passing? Why had I never brought the image of my mate up to date? My perception of him was unconnected to the real world, with its unrelenting passage of time.

As painful as it was to look time in the face, there was no way to avoid it. Little by little, reminded by my own graying hair and the lines in my face, I began to integrate my new image of us, making it more accurate and current. We were no longer teenage lovers, but our lives weren't over, either, by any means. My image of us was enriched with the maturity and wisdom that comes with experience, age, and illness.

The images you construct don't protect you from reality; they either help you or hinder you in adapting to it. Janet, an adult cardiac daughter, experienced the sorrow of losing her childhood image of her father. To Janet, Dad was powerful and strong, a man who would always be there to protect her. The reality of his heart disease forced her to confront her outdated image of him. She witnessed her forceful father, now weak and dependent, requiring a nurse's help to urinate. The new reality required that Janet grieve, and it gave her the opportunity to build an updated image of her dad.

The power of one person's images can influence another's. Edye, an earnest woman in her late thirties, related sadly that her husband, Jake, had been calling himself "damaged goods" ever since his heart attack. He was so ashamed that he even suggested Edye divorce him. Jake's image of himself had so strained their relationship that whenever Edye did anything for him, he accused her of acting out of pity.

Both Jake and Edye suffered because Jake had such a limited image of himself. Edye felt helpless, unable to convince Jake that her caring came from love and that she didn't see him as "damaged." Only Jake could transform his image. If he didn't, it would color his actions, diminish his self-esteem, influence Edye's images of him, and possibly contribute to the destruction of their relationship.

Coping with Cultural Images

In addition to personal images, we are often influenced by cultural images. Cultural images are enticing and powerful because large numbers of people accept them. The great numbers of male cardiac bypass patients, for example, help establish an image of acceptance and normalcy. In some cardiac rehabilitation programs, the bravado engendered by male cardiac camaraderie even suggests celebrity status. "Zipper chests" are recognized as a badge of courage, and cases are compared and discussed. Conversely, women having the same surgery suffer with a negative image of disfigurement and isolation. Women lack the "locker-room" opportunity for repartee and are neither prepared nor given support for their experience. No one admires their scars or offers suggestions as simple as front-closing bras, easier to negotiate after bypass surgery.

In general, it doesn't dawn on us to question the accuracy or virtue of cultural images. It's easy to brush aside our uneasiness about images seemingly accepted by everyone. They appear true and safe. But while some cultural images are correct reflections of reality, others are distorted or false. It is crucial for us to question images that don't sit right with us, that foster misconceptions and can cause harm. Examples include: heart disease is a disease of old age, heart disease only affects men, heart disease is caused by stress, heart disease means the end of normal life, including exercise and all strenuous physical and sexual activity.

Brad, a cardiac spouse in his late fifties, explained how his and Polly's lives were limited by Polly's inaccurate image of what heart disease meant for her physically. Brad first met Polly at a square dance. Although most of their interests were very different, they'd continued to square dance several times a month over the thirty-five years of their marriage. When Polly had a heart attack, she announced that her square dancing days were over, believing that the physical exertion of dancing was dangerous for heart patients.

Within a few months, Polly's physician gave her the go-ahead to resume her activities, including dancing. Despite this prescription, she was too afraid to consider it. She believed the cultural image of the debilitated heart patient. Besides, her doctor's go-ahead was only the opinion of one person. She encouraged Brad to go dancing but refused to accompany him, so Brad stayed home.

Square dancing became the thing they couldn't talk about. She felt guilty that she had made him give up dancing, and he felt guilty for wanting to go. When a counselor asked them to share their worst fear, they both had an image of Polly suffering another heart attack in the middle of a dance.

Confronting their most terrifying image, their fear lost some of its power. They decided to go to the next weekend dance. Brad reported how excited and scared they were. Brad danced the entire evening. Polly alternated between dancing and sitting out. They went home early, exhausted. But they had a wonderful time, reminiscing about the night they first met, discovering how happy they were to still have each other—and dancing, too.

Your images of life, others, and yourself can limit or free you. Start now to *examine, redefine,* and *update* your images of yourself, your mate, and your situation. Examining your images helps you to let go of the past so you can live more fully in the present.

Updating Your Images

By clinging to inaccurate and outdated images, many cardiac couples, once lovers and friends, become adversaries. Remember what you thought relationships and marriage would be like when you were young and in love? These images were often based on archetypal fairy tales (cultural and personal images)—being swept away by a handsome prince (or finding that one princess with the right shoe size) and living happily ever after. Your images probably failed to prepare you for the realities of love, relationships, and married life. And now, add a chronic, life-threatening illness to your reality.

The nature of your reality is forever different because of the heart disease. Acknowledging that the images you relied on are now shattered leaves you confused. The old images no longer fit, but you have yet to create new ones. You may understand intellectually that some of the images you had were inaccurate, but what can you believe in? Where will you find new images that reflect reality more accurately? How can you create images for your new attitudes and actions?

Mending your broken images requires time and effort, including the courageous examination of your images; a clear assessment of the accuracy of your images as compared to an objective reality; the strength to let go of the inaccurate, outdated, or self-destructive images; and a conscious effort to replace the old images with newer, healthier, more appropriate ones.

> Though painful and unsettling at times, you can trust in your ability to mend your images.

The pain of hanging on to an unrealistic image, or yearning for something that is already gone, can be eased. The cardiac crisis is a situation from which you get to look at your life's old "picture album." Nostalgia is to be expected. Capturing memories can be bittersweet. Reminiscences can stimulate fond memories and intimacy. And your images may need an overhaul. Don't burn the album; see it objectively and then look at today's picture.

This exercise is designed to help you examine images that presently motivate or direct your life in relation to your mate's heart disease. Use each set of questions as a guide. Respond with both your head and your heart. If you're writing, don't be concerned about using full sentences, making sense, or being logical. Use these questions to explore your images as fully as you can.

HEARTMATES®
GUIDE FOR EXAMINING IMAGES

- What do you recall about first visiting your mate in the hospital? In your mind's eye, see your mate and the coronary care unit as a still photo, then add sounds, smells, and movement to your image. What verbal and nonverbal messages did you receive from professional staff about your spouse's condition? See yourself then. What were you feeling, thinking, doing? Describe your feelings and the quality of communication and intimacy with your mate.

- Create an image of your mate's physical heart. As much as you can, visualize the actual damage, as well as its symbolic meaning. How is your mate's physical and emotional heart different since the onset of heart disease? Now see the healing that has occurred. Based on your image, how do you envision the long-term quality of your mate's life? Imagine yourself five years, ten years, and twenty years into the future. What effect has your mate's heart disease had on your life? How do you expect the picture will continue to change?

- What image of home and family do you have from the period of active recovery? What concerns did you have then about caring for your mate, your family, yourself? See in your mind's eye the network of communication and feelings that connected your family then. How was the family different from the way it was before the cardiac crisis? What is your image of your family now? What issues are being dealt with now by your family? What is going well for all of you?
- Look into a mirror of your past. Who were you before your mate's heart crisis? What was important to you? What was your relationship with your mate like? How was daily life organized? What were your priorities? How did you define your purpose for living? Take this past image and set it aside.
- Stand in front of the same mirror right now. Who are you today? What do you know about your strengths and limitations? How do you feel about yourself now? What is important to you today? What is your relationship with your mate like? How do you organize your daily life? What are your priorities? What is your purpose for living? Take this present image and put it alongside your past image.
- Step back far enough so you can see both images in the mirror. Visualize how being a cardiac spouse has changed you. What have you learned? How have you weathered the changes? In what ways have you taken responsibility for your recovery? How near or far are you from acceptance of what's happened to you? Have you forgiven yourself, your mate? Are you taking care of your most important needs? Which losses are you continuing to mourn? Which of your wounds have you healed and which need healing?

Purposeful examination of our images allows us to update them continually as time passes and conditions change. One of the advantages of taking stock and comparing past and present images is that you can appreciate new qualities you've developed in yourself as a response to heart disease.

Claire, who had always described herself as someone "with no head for figures," took over the family finances when her husband, Tim, was hospitalized. Tim had always paid the bills, balanced the family checkbook, and made all the crucial financial decisions. Claire, busy with her weaving, which she'd taken up seriously since her retirement, was satisfied to let Tim handle that aspect of their life. She wasn't interested and believed herself to be incompetent with numbers.

After four months of being the family banker, Claire confessed that she enjoys keeping the books. She discovered that the more she worked with figures, the more her confidence grew. Tim even called her a "crack bookkeeper." Claire occasionally still characterizes herself in the old way, but Tim just laughs. He reminds her of all the years she never even subtracted her checks in the checkbook.

Recognizing your outdated images will help you disengage from them. If you can catch yourself falling back on old images, you can learn to stop. Your mate may be willing to keep an eye out for behavior akin to your old images, to point out when you've limited yourself. Then you can consciously replace the old images with new ones that are more realistic and up to date.

What do you want your new images to be? What qualities do you want to develop? Some qualities you can use while you are healing are clarity, wisdom, love, strength, gratitude, humor, and forgiveness.

> To help you visualize and internalize the qualities you want to develop, write the quality you desire most in large letters on a three-by-five-inch card.

Use a pen or marker in your favorite color. Be playful. Add an original design, lettering and pictures that fit the quality you've chosen. Place the card where you'll see it often, where it will attract your attention. The refrigerator door, dresser top, and bathroom mirror are popular locations.

Look at the card each day. This will keep the image active in your conscious and subconscious mind. Visualize how you can express the quality in your daily life. When you stop noticing the card, you can do several things to respark your attention: move the card to a new "hot spot" or create a new card altogether, changing the coloring and design. (You also can have multiple cards up, each in a different hot spot. Rotating the cards through these hot spots every several weeks helps rekindle awareness.)

SOME IDEAS TO REMEMBER ABOUT IMAGES

- Everyone has images.
- People experience their images differently: some people summon clear visual pictures, others sense their images.
- People respond to images as if they were reality.
- Images influence understanding, attitudes, and actions.
- Images can affect physical and emotional health.
- Creating new images requires conscious effort.
- Lost, broken, invalid images need to be mourned.
- Defining yourself by an outdated image limits who you are and what you can do and be.
- Updating your images will free you to cope with and live in the present.

Forgiveness

The final step in the grieving and healing process is forgiveness—a complex, time-consuming, and difficult process for most of us. C. S. Lewis once observed that "everyone says forgiveness is a wonderful idea until they have something to forgive."

> The hardest person to forgive is often yourself, but that is where forgiveness must begin if it is to be done in earnest.

We can't truly forgive others until we forgive ourselves. The trouble is we're well practiced in criticizing and chastising ourselves, which clogs the forgiveness process and impedes healing. Once we understand and accept what has happened, we can overcome our self-recrimination and begin to have compassion for ourselves and others.

Betsy had spent most of her time since Jeff's surgery berating herself for her feelings. Her image of a good heartmate was someone who could and would ignore her own feelings and needs. Consistent focus on Jeff and gratitude for his recovery was the perfection Betsy was striving for. The more she tried to be solicitous, covering her anger and pretending concern only for Jeff, the more resentful she became. Even though she "knew she should be grateful" for Jeff's recovery, she couldn't stop feeling afraid of being abandoned. She also felt hurt that no one recognized or appreciated her needs despite the fact that she kept them to herself.

When Betsy recognized that she was responsible for keeping herself isolated, the process of forgiving herself began. As she expressed her real feelings, Betsy came to understand that she, too, had been wounded. Being gentle and forgiving toward herself set the stage for her to feel more kindly toward Jeff.

Once you recognize and accept your feelings, you will probably become more willing to confront the reality of your mate's mortality as well as your own. A longing to clean up relationships and finish "unfinished business" (to reconcile your relationships and reality) is part of forgiveness. Archbishop Desmond Tutu said, "To forgive is to abandon your right to pay back the perpetrator in his own coin, but it is a loss that liberates the victim." For many cardiac couples, liberation includes accepting mortality and imperfection of self and others.

The illusion of perfection often crumbles with the onset of heart disease. Many patients, for example, experience deep anger at the imperfection and betrayal of their bodies. Some consider divorce to punish themselves or to protect their spouses from having to live with "second-best." Like Betsy, many heartmates expect themselves to be perfectly selfless and able to provide constant caregiving. They are critical and unforgiving of themselves if they do not fulfill this expectation.

Believing that you are worthwhile and that you deserve love because you're human, not because you're perfect, is a major shift in thinking that requires real effort. To stop standing in judgment, to accept and forgive your mate and yourself for imperfections (including heart disease), is a process that takes time and hard work.

Another important task for heartmates is to accept what has happened and to forgive God or your higher power for your life circumstances. Erik Erikson suggests this wisdom: "Accept life as the only life I could ever have lived,"[17] while Phyllis Tickle connects the two tasks when she writes, "Forgiveness for how things are *is* forgiveness of God."[18] In her book, *The Last Gift of Time: Life beyond Sixty*, Carolyn G. Heilbrun expresses the gift of acknowledging mortality: "Perhaps only when we know on our pulses . . . that our time is limited do we properly treasure it."

> If you find forgiveness too difficult for now, which many heartmates do, stop trying to forgive and choose instead to focus on gratitude.

One way to focus on gratitude is to write down three things every day that you treasure in your life. After a few weeks or months, you may find yourself more at peace with a new perspective and naturally ready to forgive yourself, your mate, and the God of your understanding.

Sources of Support

No one can fully grieve and heal alone. Perhaps, paradoxically, self-care is as fundamental to healing as support from others. You need and deserve support and encouragement from yourself, as well as from others, to get through your grief.

This delicate balance between being responsible for ourselves and being connected to and supported by others may be especially difficult to manage when we are grieving. Most of us tend toward one extreme or the other. Some heartmates have internal rules that demand managing everything alone. Others feel too wounded to do very much for themselves. It is important to give yourself permission to ask others for help, and to learn to receive what's offered. On the other hand, we need to be aware of ways we can guide and be responsible for our own healing, never forgetting that we are social beings and interdependent in all aspects of our lives.

The Physical: Self-care and Support

When you use so much of your vital and emotional energy to grieve, you need to pay special attention to your physical needs to promote healing and well-being. Take vitamins. Avoid physical excesses. Be sure you get the extra sleep you require. Use soothing music to relax and induce sleep. Eat nutritious and tasty food. Include lots of fresh fruits and vegetables in your diet. Drink eight glasses of water every day, and reduce or eliminate entirely caffeine and alcohol. Wear clothes that are comfortable, cozy, and warm. Take regular breaks from your routine to stretch your muscles. Take a walk every day or stick to your regular fitness plan, but this is not the time to start a strenuous new exercise program.

Some of your physical needs require support from others. Ask family members to help with the physical tasks of managing the household that you don't have the energy to do alone. Let a friend bring in dinner and help you clean up after the meal.

When we are healing, we need to be physically touched. Stephanie Ericsson, author of *Companion through the Darkness: Inner Dialogues on Grief,* suggests that "grief tells the world that you are untouchable at the very moment when touch is the only contact that might reach you." If physical touch is not available to you at home, consider regular therapeutic massage. See your physician for any physical symptoms of stress.

If you find yourself questioning a specific activity or feeling guilty for "indulging" yourself, ask, "Will this help me heal?" Healing is not indulgent. It is essential for you to concentrate on your needs and maintain your physical well-being.

The Emotional: Self-care and Support

There are many ways to take care of yourself emotionally. Listen to beautiful music. Treat yourself to soothing teas and favorite foods. Pamper yourself. Avoid isolation. Invite help from family and friends when you feel overwhelmed. Stay away from places, people, and activities that are harsh or cold or overly demanding. Think of positive memories that evoke your feelings of pleasure and gratitude. Laugh aloud every day.

You can learn to allow yourself to be supported by others. Share your feelings with a trusted confidante. Ask yourself with whom you can talk honestly about your experiences and what you are feeling. Some people aren't able to listen in a way that is supportive. Don't waste your energy blaming or shaming yourself or them. If neither friend nor family member is available, seek emotional support from a therapist, grief counselor, or support group.

Seek out and participate in grief groups or recovery programs that encourage optimism, responsibility, and self-care. They may meet at your hospital, your church or synagogue, or your local community center.

Visit "Interactive Connections," on the Heartmates Web site <www.heartmates.com> to write your concerns and issues and read other heartmates' stories. Many have begun their search for support here over the years, building intimate and supportive friendships.

The Spiritual: Self-care and Support

Many people find their spirits replenished out in nature. Breathe deeply and inhale fresh air in your city park or along a country road to revitalize yourself. Nothing feels more nurturing than the warmth of the sun in the sky overhead and the security of the earth under your feet. Gardening has beneficial effects. Water, too, is healing; take warm baths and frequent showers. Walk by your favorite lake or, if it's near, enjoy the ocean's powerful and repetitive sound and spray.

The cardiac crisis may have clarified how much of your energy and time has been given to others. Reserve a regular time for solitude.

Give yourself downtime and silence to promote the healing of your wounded spirit.

It may be that this crisis has reawakened or deepened your religious connection. By accepting your limitations and turning to a power greater than yourself, your spirit will be nourished. Many people find that religious services and familiar rituals offer peace. Some enjoy the comfort of just sitting in a silent chapel. Others find profound value in prayer or meditation. Talk to your minister, priest, rabbi, or other spiritual leader. You know best what will help you. Make a commitment to care for your spiritual self in solitude and within your spiritual community.

Turning toward the Future

Time alone isn't enough to heal all wounds. But with the courage to face your pain and the willingness to update your images, active mourning will end. There will be clues that you have grieved enough. You can mark your progress by the fact that your life has started to return to normal. As you reorient yourself from the past to the present, more realistic images signal that you are healing.

One clear sign of recovery is commonly described as a sense of release. One heartmate realized her new freedom when whole days went by without her thinking about her spouse's heart condition or wishing for life as it used to be. Another spouse was delighted when he became aware that he was beginning to look positively to the future. He confidently made plane reservations for a vacation with his mate.

Spontaneous and genuine interest in life and others is an important indication that the crisis is behind you. I remember with pleasure a heartmate who declared enthusiastically that she was finally being released from the prison of her own pain. In the year since her husband's surgery, she had been so involved in his health that she was barely able to tolerate conversation about anything other than his condition. Her world opened like a flower as she anticipated spending meaningful time with friends and family again.

Renewed energy is another sign of your healing. During the acute crisis and often in the long months of recovery, most of your vital energy was used just to get through each day. Fatigue and exhaustion were common complaints. The return of regular eating habits and pre-crisis sleeping patterns, the easiest signs to measure, may in fact be the last physical signs of healing to occur. Now, gradually (or sometimes in dramatic bursts) you gain the physical strength to do things that for months you've been unable to consider, let alone accomplish. You'll feel renewed emotional energy, too. You may want to pick up a stimulating novel, plant a garden, make plans with friends, or involve yourself in a new project.

You will be aware of a sense of greater clarity and judgment and a growing ease in making decisions. Of course, circumstances necessitated making serious decisions long before this time, but the difference is qualitative. Recall how consuming and exhausting it felt to make decisions. Remember your confusion and frustration when you couldn't think things through? Now your ability to concentrate without undue effort has returned. Once again you can follow through efficiently.

Although progress is gradual, one day you will wake to find yourself whole again. Your present includes and integrates both the losses and lessons of your past and your newly crafted dreams for the future.

> *Lift up your eyes*
> *Upon this day breaking for you.*
> *Give birth again*
> *To the dream....*
> *Lift up your hearts*
> *Each new hour holds new chances*
> *For new beginnings.*[19]

Chapter 6 Notes

1. The significance of grieving shattered dreams was reinforced for me at a
   powerful professional workshop presented by Ted Bowman, MSW. His
   poignant and clarifying 1994 booklet, *Loss of Dreams: A Special Kind of
   Grief*, can be ordered by writing him at 2111 Knapp Street, St. Paul, MN
   55108, or by calling or faxing him at (651) 645-6058.

2. Hippocrates, *Precepts*, chapter 1, quoted in John Bartlett, *Familiar Quotations*,
   13th ed. (Boston: Little, Brown, & Co., 1955), 21. I refer you to Richard J.
   Leider's book, *The Power of Purpose: Creating Meaning in Your Life and
   Work* (San Francisco: Berrett-Koehler, 1997), in which he develops the
   idea of crisis as opportunity to focus on your "calling."

3. See Norman Cousins, *The Healing Heart* (New York: W. W. Norton, 1983)
   and his last book, *Head First: The Biology of Hope* (New York: E. P.
   Dutton, 1989).

4. Surviving the loss of their twenty-five-year-old son, who was struck by light-
   ning, is a focus of Merton P. and A. Irene Strommen's book, *Five Cries of
   Grief* (San Francisco: HarperSanFrancisco, 1993). In it they differentiate
   five kinds of pain and grief, which is useful for understanding the pain
   experienced when we deal with any major change or loss.

5. See Stephanie Ericsson's *Companion through the Darkness: Inner Dialogues on
   Grief* (New York: HarperCollins, 1993), for the most eloquent and powerful writing on grief that I have ever read.

6. After addressing cardiac rehabilitation professionals in the state of
   Washington, I was fortunate to visit the museum of the Yakima Indian
   Nation, where their values and philosophy were displayed in word and
   art. It was one of those special life experiences where beauty and truth
   were present, and so was I.

7. Rachel Naomi Remen, MD, *My Grandfather's Blessings* (New York: Riverhead
   Books, 2000); a reader-friendly book containing stories of illness, healing,
   gratitude, and other spiritual blessings. If you enjoy this book, try her
   earlier work, *Kitchen Table Wisdom* (New York: Riverhead Books, 1996).

8. Elisabeth Kübler-Ross, *On Death and Dying* (New York: Scribner Classics,
   1969, 1997).

9. Arthur W. Frank, *At the Will of the Body: Reflections on Illness* (Boston:
   Houghton Mifflin, 1991). A powerful account of a man who had a heart
   attack and cancer before he was forty. He writes honestly about his and
   his wife's experiences dealing with the illnesses, each other, and the
   healthcare system.

10. Kenneth R. Mitchell and Herbert Anderson, *All Our Losses/All Our Griefs*
    (Philadelphia: The Westminster Press, 1983).

11. Judith Lewis Herman, MD, *Trauma and Recovery* (New York: Basic Books, 1997).

12. Amelia Earhart Putnam, "Courage," quoted in John Bartlett, *Familiar Quotations*, 13th ed. (Boston: Little, Brown, & Co. 1955), 981.

13. Joan Borysenko, PhD, *Fire in the Soul: A New Psychology of Spiritual Optimism* (New York: Warner Books, 1993), 16. Borysenko cites Shelley E. Taylor, whose research and writing is about people who have readjusted well after their lives have been disrupted by misfortune. Taylor isolates three coping strategies for optimal recovery: a search for meaning in the experience, an attempt to gain mastery over the event in particular and life in general, and a recouping of self-esteem after experiencing a loss.

14. William Shakespeare, *Macbeth*, act 4, scene 3, in *Twenty-Three Plays and Sonnets*, ed. Thomas Marc Parrott (New York: Charles Scribner's Sons, 1953), 853.

15. Adapted from a broadcast on Minnesota Public Radio entitled "Positive Emotions and Health," on August 9, 1985. Presented by Norman Cousins at St. John's Hospital and Medical Center, Santa Monica, California.

16. Carl Simonton, S. Simonton, and J. Creighton, *Getting Well Again* (Los Angeles: Tarcher, 1978); and Jeanne Achterberg, *Imagery in Healing* (Boston: New Science Library, 1985).

17. Erik H. Erikson, well-respected psychiatrist and Pulitzer Prize and National Book Award winner, spent his life studying and writing about his concept of the eight stages of human development. His final book, *Vital Involvement in Old Age* (New York: W. W. Norton, 1986), challenges us all to rework the past while remaining involved in the present.

18. Phyllis Tickle, religion writer for *Publishers Weekly*, in her spiritual memoir, *The Shaping of a Life: A Spiritual Landscape* (New York: Doubleday, 2001), 217.

19. Maya Angelou, *On the Pulse of Morning* (New York: Random House, 1993), from her poem written for and read at President William Jefferson Clinton's Inaugural Ceremony on January 20, 1993, in Washington, DC.

7

Frogs Don't Turn into Princes, but Men Become Heartmates

As a male heartmate, a man in crisis, you have special concerns and needs. Coping with a mate's illness presents difficult challenges for anyone, but the situation often feels "upside-down" when the heart patient is a woman and the heartmate is a man. It can be difficult for men to adjust to this dynamic, adding further confusion, stress, and frustration to their experience.

History and culture traditionally describe men as providers and warriors, women as nurturers and caregivers. Our patterning, lifestyles, and images often mirror this description today. Men learn early, from their mothers, to expect caretaking from women. It is less common in our culture for a man to assume the role of primary caregiver.

Our traditional roles have shaped our behaviors. Men, for example, have been taught that it's strong and manly to cover their feelings. (Some men may feel comfortable revealing feelings, but most are inhibited or embarrassed about their sadness, fear, or anger.) Women in our culture have been trained to show their feelings but suppress their needs.

For you, these roles and behaviors are now being challenged, reversed, compounded. Your mate has suffered a cardiac event and she needs you for caregiving and nurturing, as well as for your more traditional roles of provider and protector. How can you perform your traditional roles, take on these new and unfamiliar roles, and recover yourself from this sudden and unexpected life change?

The answer is: with a great deal of patience, practice, and education, as well as an open heart and mind. Starting near the beginning of your story, let's begin to address your issues and needs one step at a time. In an attempt to clarify these steps, I've provided practical suggestions for navigating your caregiving experience. Watch for these highlighted tips throughout the chapter.

Unfamiliar Territory

Most cardiac events bring patients and their mates to the hospital. Once there, your partner embarks on her path toward a procedure and recovery. What are you to do?

At the outset, you will probably find yourself in the uncomfortable and foreign position of being on unfamiliar ground. You may feel like the water boy for a sports team, standing on the sidelines, hoping you'll be needed. Everyone but you has a job to do and appears busy and important. They may not even notice you standing at the nursing desk, looking lost. No one seeks you out to ask your opinion, enlist your help, or even to inform you of what's happening.

Or you may suddenly be thrown into the championship game as the quarterback. Without training or coaching you're suddenly responsible for calling the plays. Unless you have medical training, you are faced with a vocabulary of medical jargon you can barely pronounce, let alone understand. The medical team's playbook, from which you may have to make life-and-death decisions on behalf of your mate, is full of technical information difficult to decipher. Worst of all, your mate, the woman you count on as your offensive coordinator, is totally unavailable.

Staking a Claim:
Getting the Lay of the Land and Asking Directions
Your primary concern is for your mate's survival, but you also have to find your way in this new and strange environment. You'll be more

effective for your recovery and hers if you take the time to find your way around. Check out the hospital; find the family lounge, telephones, the coffee shop or cafeteria, the chapel, and the gift shop. Once you get your bearings, you'll feel more at ease.

Now you can begin to figure out the inner workings of the system. You need to become familiar with the technical language used by your partner's medical caregivers, as well as their schedules and routines. (The glossary of medical terms near the end of this book can help you "crack the code.") There's nothing you can do to change the medical team's hectic tempo, but you'll work within the system better when you understand what's going on.

Next you must get the information you need, which will probably require asking questions. You may have to play on your strengths and weaknesses. If you don't like to ask directions when you're lost driving your car, it's not hard to imagine that now, as lost as you are as your wife's heartmate, it could be difficult for you to ask questions about her condition and recovery. Your nature may be not to ask, to instead go it alone. You may believe that your competency depends on knowing, that it shows weakness to ask for directions or information. You may think or believe that you *should* be able to protect your wife and family without help from anyone.

Strive to forego the machismo, the rugged individualism, and the need to look competent at all costs. The cardiac crisis is an extraordinary situation that requires you to summon all your courage, to ask questions, to get all the information you need. Lack of information, the unfamiliar hospital setting, difficult terminology, and the precarious nature of your mate's condition contribute to the complexity of your situation. Voicing concerns and asking questions will reduce your impatience, frustration, and anxiety. Asking questions will make you a more competent provider for your mate and family.

Once you become ready to ask questions, your efforts may be frustrated by an ever-busy staff. Don't let their busyness put you off. You simply need to be as practical and task-oriented as they are. Set up a specific time (or specific times) with the nursing staff to get your questions answered. Doctors can be more tricky to speak with, but you can be successful here, too.

> Call the doctors' offices to find out when you might
> catch them at the hospital or, better yet, to make
> formal appointments to discuss your questions
> and concerns.

Your situation can be made more difficult when others, especially medical staff, are insensitive. Tim reported a meeting he had with the specialist: "The doc told me that my wife was not a candidate for bypass surgery. It felt like I was at the shop and the auto mechanic was telling me my car couldn't be fixed. I should just take it home and run it until it won't run anymore." Even when doctors are highly respected for their expertise, their bedside manner may leave a lot to be desired. It's important to be assertive, speak your needs, and ask your questions in these situations, too.

You have a right and a responsibility to access all the available data. Use the medical staff as a resource to help you find out what you, your spouse, and your family are battling, and how it will affect your lives.

> To bolster your organization, efficiency, and confi-
> dence, write your questions in a notebook or store
> them in your personal digital assistant (PDA).

After you've compiled a list of questions, decide which member of the medical team can best answer each question. Some concerns, for example, might be better handled and answered more quickly by your family doctor than your mate's cardiologist. Other questions might require the expertise of a specialist, the nursing staff, or a veteran heartmate. Write down the answers you receive in your notebook.

Most heartmates perceive the hospital staff as a lifeline of support and care for their wives. What a relief not to bear the responsibility alone! But you may also come to feel dependent on them, unsure if you should express your opinions. You may doubt the value of your input, even fear that it may be misconstrued by staff as interference. Remember that *you are the most important source of information about the patient;* you know your partner better than anyone else. Sharing your knowledge can be crucial in planning the best recovery program for her, and most hospital staff will respect and utilize your knowledge.

Put Me In, Coach
You want to feel useful and needed during your mate's hospitalization. There are things you can do directly for her that she can't do for herself and that won't interfere with the professional care she is receiving from medical staff. Moisten her dry lips, move a sheet that's pulling on a tube, or readjust a pillow. You can also ask medical staff if there are other duties you can assume. These small acts make her comfortable and express your caring. That's important for you and her.

Functioning as a knowledgeable intermediary between your wife and the professional staff can make her hospital stay easier for everyone. Communication contributes to her recovery in positive ways. Communicate for your mate when she's unable to do it for herself.

> Inform hospital staff of your wife's needs, and keep her posted about life and events outside of the hospital. This will strengthen her commitment to recover.

As the provider and family protector, your perception of success may depend on how well you solve problems. But caregiving is different; it's not about any one action or fulfilling the Mr. Fixit role. You can't fix your mate. It's about being present physically and emotionally and about listening. Your presence itself is significant to your wife. You are a symbol of stability and reality for her at a time of extreme confusion and vulnerability.

You may feel more comfortable arranging pillows and bringing her a glass of water (and these acts are helpful), but your wife also needs you just to be with her, to listen to her concerns. The support and love you offer by *being with* your wife in the hospital (and during rehabilitation at home) will contribute to her recovery far more than attempts to fix her.

It is important, too, for you to be present for yourself, to *take care of yourself*, in order to be fully present for your mate. Take time every day to "withdraw into the cave of your mind," to reduce the added stress of being unable to solve all the problems of your wife's heart disease.[1] Give yourself permission to get away for a few hours to relax, rest, and regroup. Once you've addressed your needs, you can redirect your focus and give your wife the attention she needs.

Don't forget the wisdom of airline flight attendants who remind us: "Adjust your own oxygen mask first; then assist others." One way you can adjust your own oxygen mask is by withdrawing regularly, as time and situation permit, to activities you find challenging or interesting. You might do something as simple as reading a newspaper or watching a favorite TV show. As your mate's condition stabilizes, it's not uncaring or unsupportive to attend a sporting event or to take on a favorite opponent in a game of your choice.

> Stepping out of the arena of heart disease for a few minutes or hours will allow you to release tension, clear your head, and renew your energy.

The Ultimate Juggling Act: Caring for Yourself and Others

During the acute period of a cardiac crisis, a great deal of focus is understandably on the patient. You, too, however, are in crisis, physically and emotionally vulnerable. Your daily schedule has been disrupted. You're spending many hours at the hospital. You are deeply affected by your mate's illness, and you are trying to juggle her needs with all the other demands in your life.

Giving and providing probably make you feel strong and competent, but it's important for you to pay attention to your needs. Finding ways to meet your needs as well as those of your mate can be a real balancing act. But balance between caregiving and self-care is the key to recovery for both you and your mate.

You Can Take Care of Yourself

Taking care of yourself may be a totally new concern. You may have depended on your partner to oversee much of this aspect of your life. But for now, she's not available. You are fully responsible for your own self-care.

There are many ways to take care of yourself. Some of these ways are more obvious than others. You may already do some on a regular basis. During a crisis, however, many of us forget how to take care of ourselves. The main areas of self-care are physical, mental, emotional, and practical.

Be responsible about arranging time to take care of yourself physically.

> Although your regular routine has been disrupted, be sure you are getting enough rest and that you are eating well. Take a walk at least once a day, and don't sacrifice your regular workout.

Your physical needs are more obvious and easier to plan for than your mental needs. Your mental powers, including concentration, focus, and retention, are reduced in a crisis. Be patient with yourself if you get distracted or forget details. Hospital caregivers understand your situation and most are more than willing to repeat answers or clarify information. Ask again. Use your notebook or PDA for answers as well as questions. Your "team playbook" might be an ideal place to record things you can't remember: the name of the nurse in charge, hours when hospital shifts change, phone numbers of staff you may need to contact. If you have the name of a nurse you trust, you can call her with your questions even after you've been home a while.

> Write down details; you may find them useful later.

Your need for information may be competently addressed by your hospital. Many hospitals offer educational programs that provide rehabilitation information about diet, exercise, risk factors, stress, and sexuality. These classes are to prepare the two of you for going home. Even if the focus is about your mate's recovery needs, remember that you are in crisis, too. Consider her rehabilitation prescriptions as guidelines for yourself. Think of these programs as a resource to help both of you change your lifestyles to be more heart-healthy.

Your hospital may sponsor regularly scheduled classes or programs for cardiac couples to discuss concerns that follow you home or come up later during recovery: new medications, heart-healthy food plans, smoking cessation, and lifestyle changes are a few familiar topics. Some programs include stress reduction, relaxation, and techniques for maintaining a positive attitude.

The hospital experience is the beginning of a lifelong process heralded by the initial cardiac event. Ongoing contact with the medical community is a part of life with someone who has heart disease. A positive approach is to develop respectful relationships with hospital caregivers.

The hospital is only one resource available to support you during your mate's hospital stay and recovery. You may be surprised to find that your friends and family are eager to help you both. When someone says, "What can I do?" be honest and tell them what you need. Others will seem to know exactly how to make this difficult time easier. Some might come to keep you company in the waiting room or on walks around the hospital grounds. Still others may engage you in a card game to distract your mind. In the days following hospitalization, you may have a warm meal delivered to your home. Others may come over to visit with your wife so that you aren't solely responsible, and so you can take a needed break.

When someone offers you his or her assistance, don't say, "No, no, that's okay, I'm doing fine." Learn to use this important phrase: "Yes, thank you." It is the first expression of acceptance.

It may be new for you to consider that taking care of yourself also means allowing yourself to receive from others. It's not charity; it's support. Letting your friends and relatives give to you is a gift to them, too. Giving support is a way for loved ones to express their caring, and it lets you complete practical tasks, get much-needed time-outs, and attend to your other responsibilities.

If you are going to cope successfully with the changes brought by heart disease, you need to appreciate what has happened to *you* and how you've responded. Observe yourself and your situation objectively. How have you met the challenge of your mate's life-threatening cardiac crisis? Have you allowed professionals and loved ones to support you? Are you taking good care of yourself? Take a hard look at reality, but don't sell yourself short. You may be used to getting appreciation from your wife, but her energy is now focused on her recovery. Give yourself credit for how well you've handled this complex crisis.

Acknowledge and affirm your strengths. Take credit where credit is due. Encourage yourself to continue on the road to recovery. Heartmates are awe-inspiring in crisis. Just look: You have the *courage* to ask questions and to receive support. Your *patience* lets you listen to your wife's concerns even when there are no solutions you can offer. You express *love* by being with her. Your *organizational skills* help you to be responsible at work, at home, and at the hospital, too. Each heartmate is unique and has his own qualities. Name yours, and give yourself the pat on the back you deserve.

> Look at your strengths and appreciate yourself every day.

Shifting Gears

Changed family roles and responsibilities overwhelm most heartmates as they begin to digest new demands. One of the first demands—that of "being," or simply making yourself emotionally present for your mate—can be the hardest for many male heartmates. It's common to hear a heartmate say that "just sitting at the hospital" is difficult, that he wished he could express his caring more actively. Even the most present heartmate will feel pressured and inadequate in meeting his mate's need for emotional support. Remember that your presence *is* support.

Once home from the hospital, you'll have every opportunity to "do." You bring more home from the hospital than the cards, gifts, and plants that your mate received. You also bring home the new relationship patterns that began with your mate's diagnosis. You've taken on the role of the caretaker, and this role requires you to be *and* do. Without training or preparation, you're expected to have an instant aptitude for nursing, household maintenance, even childcare. Traditional male and female roles have reversed. The woman is the recovering patient, and the man is the caregiving heartmate.

No aspect of your life is immune to this crisis. Your work schedule, leisure time, and social life have been interrupted and altered. Your primary relationship is in transition. And your personal goals and dreams, beliefs and values, are undergoing change as a result of your mate's heart disease.

The Basics: Eating and Sleeping

Basic elements of your lifestyle are the most noticeably affected early in the recovery period. At a time when you especially need nourishment and rest, you are coping with new dietary requirements and disrupted sleep. And perhaps for the first time in your life, you may be totally responsible for meal preparation and grocery shopping.

Your first serious trip to the supermarket may feel like you've been abandoned on an alien planet. Even if the layout of the store is familiar, having to find items low in fat and sodium requires familiarity with the foreign language of food labeling. Surviving the supermarket is only the beginning. The next stop is the kitchen, where the utensils are arranged according to some indecipherable code. Finding the tools and making a heart-healthy meal is stressful for all cardiac spouses. It is especially challenging for men whose experience and expertise normally lead them to the workshop, not the kitchen.

Adopting a heart-healthy food plan is the number-one concern for many couples in the early stages of recovery. Before the cardiac crisis, your responsibility may have been to sit down at the table and push away when you were finished. Now, at least for a period of time, you are the leader in the task of reshaping the family's eating habits.

Although a heart-healthy food plan is not much different than the general trend toward more nutritious eating, for the cardiac family it involves more than being fashionable or fit. It can feel like a matter of life and death. Try not to succumb to this pressure. Managing diet is practical and can be broken into simple, doable steps that can actually be a blessing when everything else feels so complicated.

Directing your mate's diet can evolve into constantly watching what she eats, counting fat grams, and monitoring salt intake. Such behavior is usually an attempt to maintain control in a situation that is overwhelming. Strive to avoid this temptation to control. Remember that there is no diet plan that will assure immortality, and there is no one way to prepare food that is right for every family.

During the transition to heart-healthy eating, communication is every bit as important as cuisine.

> Plan together and negotiate the dietary changes you and your partner want to make. Don't try to change everything at once.

Lasting change is done in small steps. Acknowledge your progress together, and celebrate the achievement of your plans.

In addition to changing dietary patterns, you will encounter changing sleep patterns. Interrupted or fitful sleep is a natural reaction to crisis and stress. Your mate is home and recovering, but you're still tense and on guard. Many heartmates report suddenly awakening during or throughout the night to make sure their recovering mates are still breathing. Though certainly not conducive to good sleep, this is par for the course. You are responding to the continuing potential for danger and will probably do so for some time.

Recovering patients often sleep fitfully, too. This change may be temporary, caused by new medications and the trauma of a heart attack or cardiac procedure. Irregular sleep or changes in your mate's sleeping patterns aren't necessarily something for you to be concerned about. Still, it may take months before you sleep peacefully again.

It's useful to know that studies have established that many of us actually need much less sleep than we think we do. Counting how many times you've awakened or how long you and your mate have slept serves only to exacerbate your worries about recovery. When you find yourself awake, use this time constructively. Pick up a magazine or book and let light reading distract and relax you. If you're restless and unable to sleep, your mate probably is, too. Give each other a back or foot rub or use the time to cuddle or talk. Chances are that after a short time, you'll fall back to sleep.

Conflicting Roles
The old pattern of your mate being present for you and your needs disappeared when heart disease appeared. You might wonder how long all her energy will be used on herself, her disease, her symptoms, her recovery. You've been left to fend for yourself without a word of explanation or a promise that the tables will turn again. Almost as quickly as you think such thoughts, you feel guilty. She might have been lost to me forever; how can I think of myself? But the thoughts don't go away. They are normal.

Similarly, female patients often have difficulty accepting or enjoying being taken care of. They, long defined by their role of caretaker, find it difficult to let go. These women may respond to caring with irritability, anger, impatience, and criticism.

You and your mate need to discuss how your lifestyles and relationship roles are changing due to heart disease and how to negotiate these adjustments in your lives. Without communication, there is potential for misunderstanding, conflict, and hurt feelings.

Stan, known to his family and friends as the strong, silent type, struggled to express his caring and love to his wife. He had never been effusive, and, like many men of his generation, he was uncomfortable articulating his feelings and assuming the role of caregiver.

Stan loved Jean dearly. After her heart attack, he showed his love, concern, and effort to be a good caregiver by doing all the household chores after his regular long hours at work. He was particularly proud of his vacuuming. Jean didn't appear to appreciate Stan's efforts or to realize that his cleaning was a way to say "I love you."

As soon as she felt well enough, Jean resumed vacuuming and her other chores. Stan felt frustrated with Jean's perfectionism and afraid that she was pushing herself too fast. Mostly, however, he felt useless and incompetent.

Jean, needing to test her own fitness after her heart attack, did what she knew best: reclaimed her role by taking over her household tasks. Because the traditional feminine role of caretaker was familiar to her, Jean felt uncomfortable being cared for and guilty about Stan doing both "their jobs." In her haste to recover, she failed to appreciate her heartmate, Stan.

With all our society's sophisticated technology, we don't communicate much differently from the way we did when we lived in caves. Too often we rely on single-syllable grunts rather than telling each other how we feel. Since they did not talk about their thoughts or feelings, Jean had no way to know that Stan was expressing love and care for her by taking over her tasks. Stan didn't understand that Jean was eager to resume her chores because she felt helpless, stripped of her habitual roles and activities.

Communication aids understanding. Whether differences between men and women are caused by hormones or homemaking doesn't matter. What's important is that men and women understand and appreciate their inherent or learned differences so that the differences don't distance them from one another. How might Stan have felt if Jean had explained her feelings of discomfort, helplessness, and guilt? Her role was to take care of their nest, and she was ashamed to see him vacuuming and cooking. And how might Jean have responded had she heard from Stan that she'd undermined his ability to do things for her, and that he felt useless and unappreciated?

> Recognize that you and your mate are different. Communication about feelings and roles can bridge these differences.

It's easy to slip into criticism, bitterness, and alienation when both partners are experiencing changing, relinquished, and resumed responsibilities. One recovering heart patient explained to her friend, who had come over to assist with the laundry, "Mick 'helped' me by doing the laundry, but I saved these loads for you. He washes it all together, he fills the machine too full, and he dries everything in the dryer. Men just don't understand about the laundry."

Communication can help you avoid the pitfall of criticism. By communicating with each other you can learn about areas of need, skill, and weakness. Perhaps more importantly, communication can lead you to better understand and appreciate your differences, preventing bitterness and alienation.

Working Out Work

Work and career will be a concern for you and your mate. Your mate might be able to return to her old job, but her heart disease could also require her to retire or change vocation. Talking about career matters is personal, stressful, and scary. You may hesitate to raise the subject or express your opinions about the matter because you don't want to add stress to an already difficult situation. Keep the lines of communication open anyway.

Your efforts and input are valuable to your mate as she deals with the work issue and the decision-making process. Avoiding it won't really alleviate stress or make the issue disappear. Ignoring such a sensitive topic may become a bigger problem than confronting it head on. Once you make the effort to communicate, you might be relieved to find that your mate has questions and concerns similar to yours. Together you can confront the career issues you are both facing.

Although you may have been the primary breadwinner in your family, the delay of your mate's return to work, restrictions on the hours she is able to work, or her early retirement can add pressure to your lives during the recovery period and beyond. You may wonder how you'll ever again afford your lifestyle. You worry about medical bills piling up. The pre-cardiac plans you shared for early retirement or a timely retirement may be lost. Your fears and concerns can seem limitless.

Your mate's job probably meant more to her than the money she earned. It provided a sense of empowerment, independence, and service. Your mate may be afraid of becoming uncomfortably dependent on you if she doesn't earn her own money. She may be grieving other work-related losses as well. What can she do that would be as fulfilling, as satisfying, as her job? What about the friendships she enjoyed with her longtime coworkers?

> Take time to talk about your feelings and make decisions together about the changes in your careers, economic plans, and leisure time.

Even if your feelings on these subjects aren't similar, two heads are better than one. Explore creative ways to adjust to your new lifestyle and its demands on you. Seek professional counsel if you and your mate can't talk about work-related issues.

Downshifting

Your social and leisure activities have been affected by the cardiac event and your new cardiac lifestyle. Previously simple decisions, like whether to see a movie or play doubles tennis, become major issues in adjusting to this new lifestyle. You want to protect your mate's health, but at the same time you need to maintain your friendships and social interests.

You may question your partner's motivation, feel impatient, or even harbor resentment that she isn't improving more rapidly. Heartmates often wonder: "Why is she so tired? Why is she still depressed? Why isn't she feeling better by now?" The reality, however, is that the patient needs time and psychological space to integrate the many changes resulting from heart disease. You will probably have to alter your expectations during recovery. Crossing the bridge from active recovery to full recovery takes time, effort, and patience.

Bruce planned a trip to Disney World for his recovering wife, children, and grandchildren, thinking that a vacation would lift Mattie's spirits. Mattie's recovery was happening in fits and starts, with her feeling down some days, wanting only to sit at home, and her feeling more energetic and outgoing other days. Bruce came to understand that his anxiety about Mattie's depression, as well as his desire to speed the recovery process and return to a normal life, were the impetus for what would have been a strenuous trip for all of them. To Mattie's relief, Bruce canceled the reservations and dealt with his and their family's disappointment.

There isn't anything you can do to speed up the recovery process, but there are ways to adapt to it. During this active recovery, talk with your mate to establish realistic expectations. Doing so will help you interact with each other, friends, and family in ways that work and are satisfying. You might have to ask family and friends to be flexible in accommodating your needs. Hopefully they'll be understanding and tolerant. What were once shared nights at the bowling alley, for example, can be replaced by a quiet evening watching movies and munching salt-free popcorn.

As a heartmate, your days will come to feel normal more quickly than your mate's, especially once you return to the routine of work. You may find yourself wanting to work longer hours and spend more time with friends. But what about your recovering mate? As the weeks of recovery become months, planning time apart becomes important, a way to respect your own individuality and your wife's.

It's normal and healthy to want to reclaim your work life. It's a part of you that needs attention. Your mate, too, needs to feel empowered and in control of her life. Talk with her about your need to work. She probably feels a need to reclaim activities, tasks, and roles that you took over when she couldn't do them for herself.

It's also normal and healthy to want to reclaim your recreational life. But you may think that the seriousness of your mate's heart disease precludes your own recreation and fun. You may not have the same enthusiasm for activities and projects you once did. Or you might simply wonder when it's appropriate to return to your hobbies, activities, meetings, and friendships. You probably fear social criticism, worrying about being seen in public having a good time when your mate has suffered a heart attack and is at home recovering. You wonder if you'll appear insensitive, uncaring, or selfish.

You might, but the choice about when you resume activities is an individual and personal matter between you and your mate. It's crucial that *you* be involved in something besides work and caring for your recovering mate. Before your mate's cardiac event, you took the structure of your life for granted; returning to that order will increase your sense of control and safety. Whether you work in the yard, rearrange your tool room, or go fishing or golfing, *taking time for yourself* every day will help you and your mate heal.

In addition to your guilt, doing your own thing may, at first, produce anxiety. As you wean yourself gradually from habits that began as caregiving at the hospital (when your wife was vulnerable and unable to take care of herself), your anxiety will diminish.

Talk with your mate every week to plan time apart from each other; renegotiate events and time apart as recovery unfolds. Start by leaving your mate alone for a short time: meet a friend for breakfast or a racquetball game, or go out for a run. Work up to more lengthy periods of separation. Maintaining your interests is essential for your recovery and will be paramount in restoring a healthy balance in your relationship.

> Say no to guilt and anxiety. Your healing depends on you resuming activities that nurture you.

The Emotional Poker Game

During the initial phases of the cardiac crisis, it's normal for you to feel numb and shaky, to have trouble concentrating and difficulty staying focused on conversations. These are typical reactions. Throughout the early phases of the crisis, limit yourself to addressing only those tasks and decisions that absolutely cannot wait.

As the numbness wears off, you'll become aware of your feelings, especially fear. The most compelling of your terrors is that you'll lose your mate. This is the fear of loss and abandonment that is common to everyone and heightened in those experiencing crisis and trauma. In the acute crisis even small things feel disproportionately threatening.

Your fears may be expressed in various ways, including loss of appetite, trembling, shallow breathing, edginess, or insomnia. Fear paralyzes some people, makes others withdrawn, causes still others to become jittery or restless, irritable or angry. Everyone has a hard time coping with the unknown and the threat of potential loss.

Learning to live with uncertainty is the heartmate's greatest challenge.

> *There is no certainty;*
> *there is only adventure.*
> *Even stars explode.2*

Knowing that your mate is under the care of competent professionals may reduce your fear, but until your mate is home and recovering for more than a few weeks, it's normal for your fear to surface.

The first six months of recovery is a particularly difficult adjustment period for you individually and as a couple. While there is much to be grateful for, transition is ever present. Your life continues to change, dealing you uncertainty on a regular basis. The changes may be both obvious and subtle.

At the onset of the cardiac crisis, there were major ruptures in your relationship. You were separated from each other physically and emotionally, with one in the hospital, the other at home. Limited hospital visits, protecting your wife from stress, and disguising your feelings of fear and worry disrupted communication and distanced you from her. You each may have retreated to protect yourselves, too.

Some couples carry their protective emotional distance (which can manifest in physical distance as well) into recovery and beyond. Although you may not be aware of the dynamic, it takes a lot of energy to keep your poker face on, to camouflage your feelings and maintain distance. In the long run, your energy is depleted, and it's easier to fold than to be courageous and persevere with your dealt hand.[3] Intimacy and honesty will help each of you and your relationship to heal.

One way to improve communication and understand how each of you feels about issues and concerns is to express feelings regularly. Here is an exercise that may help:

> Set aside two minutes each day. In that time, tell your mate one thing that you are feeling. Ask her to share one feeling with you. No solutions are allowed. No responses are required of either of you. Just listen to each other.

See chapter 8 for more information about communication and intimacy.

It is natural to push away unwanted feelings during the height of the emergency. Although she may not say anything, your wife is probably experiencing feelings and reactions similar to yours. She is coping with the physical adjustments to heart disease and with the emotional effects as well. Both of you need permission to have, not hide, all the feelings you are feeling, including the "negative" ones (feelings are just feelings; they are neither positive or negative, though they may feel this way).

The Fear and Anxiety Cards

Recognize what your feelings are. In the heartmate's emotional poker game, the royal flush is dealt by the king of darkness—fear. The unexpected threat of losing the person most precious to you, the person on whom you've depended, causes deep fear, anxiety, and even terror. These emotions don't just go away, even when full recovery is the expected prognosis.

We live in an instant age, and we take for granted a speed unheard of in earlier times: jet travel, twenty-second sound bites, faxes, the Web. So it's not surprising that we expect ourselves to heal from the cardiac crisis quickly, efficiently, and perfectly. But even full recovery does not mean the absence of fear; most people continue to experience fear for years, though it diminishes over time. Your body learned to respond to the crisis with anxiety reactions, and it will continue to respond this way for a long time, unable to differentiate between a cough and a cardiac arrest.

*A*lmost ten years after my spouse's heart attacks and bypass surgery, I was surprised to find my fear close to the surface. It was a beautiful August afternoon, and he was on the golf course. I had just come in from weeding my garden when the phone rang. Answering it, I heard an unfamiliar voice, "Hello?" "Yes," I responded. I could already feel anxiety churning deep inside.

"This is Mrs. Jones from the golf course," she said. I knew my worst fantasy was about to come true. "Yes," I said again, trying to hurry her telling me the dreadful news. The uncertainty was devastating. I was sure that I had lost my mate. She continued, "We're wondering if you and your husband would like to join our bowling league this fall?"

I thought I had totally recovered from my fear and anxiety; after all, it had been years. The fact is, anytime something unfamiliar and unexpected happens, we will feel residual fear and anxiety. The heartmate wound scars over, yet it remains just beneath the skin.

Anxiety may be expressed as a physical symptom in the body (sleeplessness, headaches, lack of appetite, tense and aching muscles) or an overwhelming feeling of helplessness. The first best step in dealing with anxiety is admitting to yourself that you are afraid. For most people, the fear is about losing their mate. Once you've ascertained that you're afraid, you can use logic to help you process and deal with it. Ask yourself about the evidence for your anxiety, and then act appropriately. What is the real danger in this situation? Are there other symptoms beyond the cough you hear? What is your wife's assessment of the situation?

Many men try to reduce or avoid their anxiety by keeping busy, doing something to feel more in control.

> Find ways to relieve your anxiety and simultane-
> ously protect your spouse.

Probably the most common way is to gather information about heart
disease and recovery, but you can take other measures that will help
you feel more secure and prepared. Visit your local fire station to
introduce yourself to the paramedics in your area. They may be able
to code your address screen on the 911 program to indicate that your
wife is a heart patient.

If your wife has a severe and increasingly debilitating condition,
such as congestive heart failure, then chronic anxiety may be the
norm for you. In such cases it can be helpful to seek advice and
treatment from your physician in addition to the anxiety-coping
methods shared here.

Anger: The King of Cards

Another emotion hidden behind your poker face is probably anger.
Although feelings are just feelings and feelings aren't rational, you
may have valid reasons for your anger. You may be angry at medical
staff or at your family for failing to recognize your needs. You may
be angry at something as vague and abstract as your wife's genetic
predisposition for heart disease. You may feel indignant about how
your life has changed, and about the additional responsibility you
have taken on to be both provider and caretaker. If you're used to
relying on your wife to meet many of your emotional needs, you
may resent her neglect.

Recognize your feelings of anger and monitor your expression of
it and other emotions. Unrecognized and unexpressed anger
doesn't go away. It "comes out sideways" or sits in layers, waiting to
be dealt with. If left untreated, unexpressed anger will harden into
rage and resentment.

Expressing anger to your wife will not endanger her health.[4] There are
safe ways to express anger, with direct communication being the most
effective. Although there is no guarantee that you'll get what you

need, using your anger constructively to determine and express your needs tends to help you release it.

> Tell your mate when you're feeling frustrated or angry. Find safe, physical outlets: run, swim, or hit any kind of ball as hard as you can.

Sadness and Guilt: The Low Cards
We take our lives for granted until something threatens our security. Then we experience enormous feelings of loss. *It is absolutely normal for you to feel sad, disappointed, and depressed.* In addition to anger, these are some of the very human feelings of grief. As you yearn for times past, for your secure, pre-cardiac life, you are grieving what you've lost.

Our society tends to honor and respect those who seem strong and decisive, appearing to feel no pain. You may be tempted to hurry through, minimize, or deny your own sadness. But grieving is human and necessary for healing. We each grieve at our own pace, and feeling sad is not a sign of weakness, craziness, or failure. Give yourself the time you need to recover from the emotional trauma of the cardiac event and all the changes that have occurred since. Treat yourself with the same generosity of spirit that makes you tolerant of the time your wife needs to recover from the physical trauma she has lived through.

Guilt is a tricky card in the deck of the heartmate's feelings. Many men assume guilt for their mate's heart disease. They think they should have been able to prevent it and feel guilty that they didn't. Even as our culture moves toward gender equality, we hold on to the belief that good men are successful providers and protectors.

Maintain perspective when you draw this particular card. There is no way that you could have protected your wife from suffering a cardiac event. Wiring an alarm system or installing special door and window locks may protect against intruders, but you have no special skills or divine powers to protect your wife from heart disease.

There are many other things that trigger guilt in heartmates. You probably feel guilty when you want your needs met. You might feel guilt, for example, when you want your wife to be healthy again, to reestablish her responsibilities, or to be present for the sexual aspect of your relationship. You can experience guilt for taking your mate and her health for granted. And then there's always the guilt of wanting to return to your own normal life activities.

Some men feel guilty about being queasy or turned off at seeing their mate's incision or scar after open-heart surgery. (Men's scars, ironically, are often considered handsome by many in our culture. Men's scars may be deemed a "red badge of courage," symbolizing bravery. But not so for women, whose bodies are supposed to be perfect.) Logically, you can tell yourself not to feel the way you do, that the chest scar from open-heart surgery is not a disfigurement; but logic doesn't always change what we feel. Hiding disgust and the guilt that comes with it behind a poker face will not help, either; expressing how you feel probably will.

> It always helps to voice your feelings. If your guilt, sadness, anger, or fear will hurt your mate or add to her burden during recovery, try writing your feelings down and keep that writing in a private place. Or, share your feelings with a friend you can trust.

Sharing with a Trusted Friend

Working through a crisis is a highly personal experience. At times, solitude might be exactly what you need to sort through your varied feelings and whirling thoughts. But too much isolation is detrimental to recovery. If you hold everything tight to your chest and never show your hand, your healing will only be partial.

It's important to your healing to seek out others with whom you can share your experience, your story. Sharing your story will help you understand and release what you've gone through and what you're going through now. It will also provide you support, reduce the weight of your worries, and guide you toward acceptance and healing. Be sure to choose a person who can listen, someone who will be a witness and not a judge.

> Your confidant should be someone willing and able to hear your feelings without being afraid. He or she should also be someone who will respect your confidentiality.

Charlie called Fred, his old hometown pal, a couple months after Robin's heart attack and subsequent procedure. He was relieved to hear Fred's voice and his concern. Fred was coming to the city and thought they should get together. Charlie agreed, looking forward to an evening away from Robin and eager to be with a friend with whom he could just be himself.

When they met, Charlie told Fred how scared he had been, and how frustrated and guilty he felt because Robin's recovery was taking longer than Charlie had expected. It felt good laying everything on the table and having Fred validate how strong he'd been when Robin needed him. They decided to get together regularly when Fred returned to the city, and Charlie went home to Robin feeling much better.

Many heartmates naturally select family members as confidants. But family members might not be the best choices available to you. While your family knows you best and longest, they don't have first-hand knowledge about what you've experienced. You may not have the kind of supportive relationships in your family that you need right now. Family members may also be too close to the event, experiencing their own difficult feelings, to be present for you. Family members can be present and supportive in other ways, including meal preparation, childcare, or even financial support.

Ideally, your confidant will be someone able to identify with your story. There's great comfort in hanging out with a group of male heartmates. Reaching out to others who have lived through similar cardiac experiences can help you and them heal, providing much-needed acceptance, understanding, and validation. Attend educational and support programs at your local hospital or community center (with your spouse and by yourself).

Unfortunately, at times, trusted confidants may not be around to listen when you need to share deep feelings. During these times, consider talking to your minister, priest, rabbi, or other spiritual leader. You can also make an appointment to speak with a professional counselor. Twelve-Step meetings provide a supportive environment for telling your story and sharing your feelings, too. They are confidential, and groups such as Al-Anon and CoDA (Codependents Anonymous) focus on coping with feelings and relationships.

The toughest part of your recovery may be realizing and accepting that you can't do it all. Traditional masculine behavior—to be strong, silent, and handle everything alone—doesn't work in the extraordinary circumstances of a cardiac crisis. Reach out to family, friends, and other supportive people for help. Find a way to tell your story.

Taking Care of Your Own Business

I asked male heartmates what the hardest thing was for them when their mates first came home from the hospital. Here are some typical responses: "Trying to keep her from working too hard. Preventing her from doing work around the house. Making sure she took her medications on time. Maintaining a strict schedule for her exercise. Keeping her from moving ahead too fast. Not letting her do too much."

Although I knew that most female heartmates tend to be overly protective of and overresponsible for their mates, I was surprised to hear echoes of the same attitude from male spouses. As with your female counterparts, you male heartmates often cross the line from caregiving to caretaking.

Your caregiving begins out of love, but fear can quickly motivate caretaking. That fear is often experienced as an uncomfortable feeling of helplessness. Because you can't change the fact that your wife has heart disease, you compensate by taking charge, by becoming overresponsible for your mate, her behavior, her recovery.

Heartmates who caretake are trying to control the uncontrollable. They come to believe that their mate's recovery is in their hands. It's not. *You neither caused her heart disease, nor do you have the power to cure it.* Your caretaking will be detrimental to her recovery, your recovery, and your relationship.

Heart patients can be frightened by their mates' pressuring them to do less. They wonder if you know something the doctors didn't tell them. They fear that they might be worse than they thought. But the greatest consequence to your mate, stemming from your caretaking, is a loss of confidence and responsibility for herself. She will wonder if she's become incompetent, worthless. She may even come to resent you for implying that she is helpless.

Power struggles are often the result of caretaking, and they are legendary among cardiac couples. The more you try to get her to do less, the more she will attempt to do. Control is met with resistance, and the pattern spirals. The more you are overresponsible for her, the more she resists. The more she resists, the more unappreciated you feel for the solutions you're suggesting.

What your mate really needs is to know that you love, respect, and support her. Some of the most supportive, loving, and respectful actions you can take are simple.

> Show your strength and caring by listening to your
> wife without telling her what to do or how to do it.

You can let her know you're willing and ready to assist her with tasks, diet, and other aspects of recovery, should she need and want your help. One of the simplest, yet most loving and powerful, acts of support is hugging your mate and telling her that you love her.

You can't live your mate's life, do her recovery, or keep her alive. No matter how much you love her, you cannot take away her basic responsibility for herself. Besides, the more energy you focus on her behavior and her recovery, the less attention you can pay to your own.

Getting in Touch Again

Many people think of intimacy in its most limited definition—sex. But intimacy, an essential component of recovery, needs to be understood more broadly. In his novel, *A Soldier of the Great War,* Mark Helprin poignantly expressed the human dilemma of love and mortality in a dialogue between two soldiers:

> *"I see that the most beautiful thing between a man and a woman is not the consummation of their love, but, simply, their regard for one another."*
>
> *"That may be so, but you probably can't know it until you're condemned to die."*
>
> *"You're always condemned to die. It's just a matter of timing."*[5]

Being in recovery together can be an opportunity to express your regard for each other. Many couples find their awareness heightened, their hearts expanded. What you took for granted before heart disease is now experienced as precious. You may come to appreciate each other more and find new ways to express your love.

You both need to give and receive physical comfort. Holding hands, walking arm in arm, hugging and kissing, cuddling and spooning all are warm ways to get back "in touch" with your partner again.

Don't change pre-cardiac sleeping arrangements. The physical separation when she was in the hospital was hard on both of you. Continue sleeping in your bed together. Each knowing that the other is there, reaching out to touch each other, is comforting.

Although sex may be on hold for a time, there's no reason to stop being intimate. Beauty and love belong to everyone if we dare to see them and live them. What is special is you and your mate being together the way you really are. Physical caring is expressed throughout life and all over the world in as many different ways as there are people. Your renewed discovery of each other, your soft, quiet embrace, may mean more to each of you now than you ever imagined.

If you're like many people, you were probably taught that sex is a private matter, so it's difficult for you to talk about it. Here, then, is an opportunity for you to be courageous. Expanding your intimacy includes telling each other how you feel. Tell your mate how glad you are that she survived the cardiac crisis, how lonely it was without her, how wonderful it is to hold her in bed again, that you miss being close to her, that you love her. Talking about sex begins with small steps. Tell her what you want and need, and ask her how she feels, and what she wants and needs. From this gentle and mutually respectful act, you can create your physical intimacy.

What about Sex?

Attitudes about sex and the level of sexual activity are subject to many influences, including age, gender, and health. Male heartmates have specific questions and expectations about sex. Part of your journey through the recovery period is trying to understand how sex fits into the "new normal," your life with a mate who has heart disease.

The most common questions include: Will having sex hurt or endanger her? Why is she so disinterested in sex, and in me? Does she still care about me? Will her attitude change as time goes on? How much is she affected by heart disease and how much by the normal aging process?

Let's begin with answers about the physical aspects of sex. While physical recovery is unique to each person, the medical literature indicates that by six weeks after a cardiac event most heart patients can resume their normal activities, including sex. It takes about that long for the heart to heal after a heart attack, perhaps slightly longer for breastbones and incisions to heal after open-heart surgery. After a balloon angioplasty or a cath procedure, if your wife has not had a heart attack, physical activities, including sex, are restricted for twenty-four hours so the puncture site can safely close.[6]

When we look at the emotional dimension of a cardiac event in relation to sexuality, the picture gets more complicated. Some women are not interested in sex because they are depressed. *Depression is normal for patients and heartmates* off and on for as much as a year after a cardiac event. People who are depressed lack energy and are disinterested in all kinds of activities, including sex, that were normal and enjoyable for them before the crisis.

Some men respond to emotional crisis with physical impotence. If that happens to you for more than a few weeks, talk with your doctor about how it can be treated. Talk with your wife, too. Sharing with each other may help to release feelings that have increased your stress. Remember, it takes two to tango, and sex is basic in the dance of relationship.

Your mate may be apprehensive about sex, too. She may want to hide her body from you after surgery because she feels disfigured and ugly. She may believe she's undesirable, no longer attractive to you. She might be anxious and afraid of sex, even after she has been assured it is okay to return to her normal, active lifestyle. Again, communication is the key to true and comfortable intimacy. Once fears are expressed, no longer hidden in shameful silence, you both may feel lighter, less burdened, and more connected to each other.

Recovery is also a time when both your sexual needs may be in flux along with other, deeper changes: priorities, values, meaning. You may not have noticed that your sexual desire or activity was changing gradually as you aged until the cardiac crisis brought it into focus. Although it may seem like a dramatic shift, it's more likely that your awareness has been heightened by your recent experience, where everything seems different and difficult.

Your shifting sexual relationship is only one of the challenges you face together. This time of your life has the potential to be the richest and fullest yet experienced. Celebrate your time together, one day and one touch at a time. Remember, the road to success is always under construction.

TOP TEN REMINDERS FOR MALE HEARTMATES

1. You have needs in the cardiac crisis: for information, to be needed, for support.
2. You have a right to information. It will help you make informed decisions and reduce your anxiety and feelings of helplessness.
3. Take good care of yourself. You are in crisis and recovery, too.
4. Ask for and let yourself receive support. Isolation will impede your recovery.
5. Make plans for lifestyle changes with your mate.
6. Fear, depression, guilt, sadness, and anger are normal emotional responses to the cardiac crisis and during recovery.
7. Share your feelings and tell your story to another person you can trust: a close friend, other heartmates, your spiritual leader, or a competent professional.
8. Recognize and be tolerant of differences between you and your mate.
9. Talk to each other; touch each other.
10. Celebrate life today!

Chapter 7 Notes

1. John Gray, PhD, "Men Go to Their Caves and Women Talk," *Men Are from Mars, Women Are from Venus* (New York: HarperCollins, 1992), 30–31. This popular book articulates differences between men and women, offering practical suggestions about what to do to bridge the divide. Heart disease highlights how different husbands are from their wives, and how those differences affect recovery for the patient, heartmate, and the couple.
2. It's normal to wish for security and constancy. Roberto Assagioli (1888–1974), Italian physician and founder of psychosynthesis, reminds us of the permanence of change.

3. Chapter 8 of this book is about healing the cardiac couples' relationship. There are two major sections in the chapter: one focuses on communication, the other focuses on sexuality.

4. See "Anger: The Ogre" in chapter 3 of this book for guidance in the healthy expression of anger for cardiac couples.

5. A poignant passage from Mark Helprin's novel, *A Soldier of the Great War* (New York: Harcourt, Brace, 1991), 421.

6. If you want to read more about sexuality, see the second half of chapter 8, "Re-pairing the Heartmate Connection," in this book. In my questionnaires to male cardiac spouses, gathered prior to writing this chapter, more men responded to the question about sex than to any other question. Most indicated that their sex life was "worse" since their wife's cardiac event.

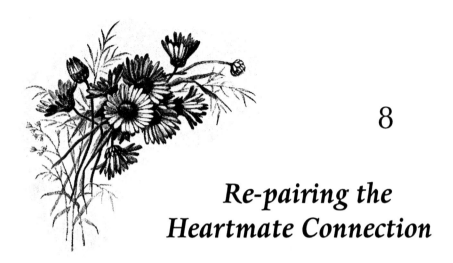

8

Re-pairing the Heartmate Connection

The love bond, symbolized by the heart in song and literature, is threatened or tested by the cardiac crisis. This connection was interrupted during your mate's stay in the hospital. Once he returned home, each of you remained isolated as you tried to protect each other from undue suffering and stress.

Heart disease affects *all* relationships, including strong, loving ones. According to author and social scientist Edward J. Speedling, when a physical trauma of the magnitude of a cardiac event occurs, the love relationship is challenged. "The act of healing," Speedling states, "cannot be complete until the social and emotional bonds that the illness disrupted are revitalized."[1]

The cardiac crisis draws some couples closer together, resulting in greater support and intimacy. Many heartmates' devotion to each other is enhanced. You may be keenly aware of how much you cherish and need your mate. For other cardiac couples, the trauma pulls them apart, intensifying already existing conflicts. You may now see even more clearly the flaws in your relationship. Unfortunately for some, the disease creates the final rift in an already strained relationship.

It's not fair to blame all the imperfections in your relationship on heart disease. Chronic illness has a powerful effect on patterns in your relationship that were established long ago. Conversely, the quality of your relationship affects your physical and emotional recovery.

One can't assume that because the patient has physically recovered, the relationship is automatically healed. In order for your relationship to mend, you and your mate need to recover individually and put effort into healing your partnership. At the very least, a relationship needs to be flexible enough to adapt to a new reality that includes heart disease, putting the illness in its place.

Heart disease can be the catalyst for a more intimate relationship. Repairing the heartmate connection goes hand in hand with your recovery. Honest confrontation of the changes in your relationship can deepen your love connection.

Communication between Heartmates

The value of good communication is generally recognized in our society. The acute crisis has undoubtedly affected your communication patterns. For some couples, the disruption is minor, like assuming a quieter tone of voice. For others, more dramatic changes occur, ranging from an overly polite stance to no communication at all.

Caring communication is essential for healing a wounded relationship. Begin by looking realistically and honestly at the changes in your communication. Examining your communication does not mean that you are under any obligation to do anything different. Use the following checklist to observe "what was" and "what is" in order to evaluate your present communication with your mate. (As you answer the questions, keep in mind how you would have responded before heart disease.)

HEARTMATES®
COMMUNICATION EVALUATION CHECKLIST

Yes	No	
___	___	1. Has your tone of voice or your manner of talking to your mate changed?
___	___	2. Are you more careful, measured, about the words you use when you talk to your mate?
___	___	3. Are there unusually long silences when the two of you are together?
___	___	4. Is it difficult to keep conversation going between you?
___	___	5. Do you direct conversation away from yourselves and toward others?
___	___	6. Is your television on more often than before the cardiac crisis?
___	___	7. Are you less expressive of your feelings?
___	___	8. Are you more silent about your concerns?
___	___	9. Do you feel more lonely, isolated, misunderstood?
___	___	10. Do you talk regularly about daily routines, long-term plans, and dreams?
___	___	11. Do you discuss taboo issues (life and death, sex, finances, love) since the cardiac crisis?
___	___	12. Are you generally satisfied and emotionally supported by communication with your mate?

This evaluation helps you see your communication from a new perspective. If your answers reveal major changes in communication, ask yourself if these changes are positive or negative. Directly comparing your communication before and after the cardiac event can be useful. If you find that your communication is more circumscribed, less spontaneous than it was before heart disease, for example, you can choose to change it.

Some people find it difficult to be objective and specific about their lives. If the evaluation doesn't help you assess the quality of communication with your mate, consider visualization. This may help you recognize the strengths and limitations in your pattern of communication. It may also increase awareness of how images impressed during your mate's crisis may be getting in the way of healing your relationship.

Imagine the heartmate bond as a cord that connects you and your mate. Picture, for a moment, the symbolic flow of communication between your two hearts. How much moves through the cord? What color is the communication moving through the cord? Is the color warm or cool? Is the communication thick or thin, sluggish or flowing smoothly? Is the cord's passageway tight and clogged, or is it clean and open to the flow of communication? Does your image evoke a picture of communication that is open, severed, or somewhere in between?

For some couples, the cardiac experience provokes serious soul-searching and sharing. Other couples become self-conscious and estranged, and in the most extreme cases, they live like strangers. But most of us communicate somewhere in between, depending on the day, outside support, level of illness, and other factors.

> The evaluation checklist and the visualization exercise will provide information about your pattern of communication. The purpose is for each of you to break through your isolation and make progress in healing your relationship.

If you discover major changes in communication since the cardiac crisis, decide whether the way you are communicating is keeping you distant or bringing you closer together. You can choose to change the way things are. Remember, take one step at a time. Agree on specific changes and evaluate how you're progressing.

Myths to Dispel

The way you communicate is further influenced by myths. A myth is a culturally learned belief that affects how you act and how you feel. Beliefs, even if they are myths, form our reality. As a heartmate you are particularly vulnerable to three myths that impede communication. Strive to recognize, dispel, and replace these myths. The result will be communication that is free and rewarding for both of you.

Myth 1: It Is Better for the Patient If You Don't Communicate Your Concerns and Fears

Protection is the motivation underlying the myth of sheltering secrecy. When your mate was in the hospital, there were rules and guidelines defining what he could and could not handle. Common sense also guided your interaction with the patient. Your love for your mate and desire to protect him merged with these rules and guidelines. As a result, you may have come to believe that it's best not to worry the patient with concerns of any kind, ever.

During recovery, you have a new challenge: to adapt communication and intimacy to a relationship complicated by a chronic illness, to share as openly and honestly as recovery permits. The myth of protective secrecy, however, often follows heartmates home and is acted out well into recovery. One man proudly announced that he was protecting his wife so well that she had no inkling he'd taken a second job to meet their medical expenses. Another spouse struggled alone with her teenage son's drug abuse, fearful of the consequences of involving her recovering mate.

Patients' reactions to protection vary, but most feel controlled, insignificant, and distrusted. Finding out that Lulu had made important financial decisions without asking for his input, for example, Frank's rage erupted. "For thirty years of marriage, I was good enough to take care of it," Frank asserted. "One little heart attack, and now I'm a nincompoop with no brain. I can't do anything around here," he shouted and stormed out of the house.

> *What loneliness is more lonely than distrust?*
> George Eliot

The fact is, there is no proof that avoiding communication is beneficial to a heart patient. It is certain that concealing your concerns increases the distance between you and your mate and intensifies feelings of distrust, loneliness, and abandonment. Your relationship will weaken without open, quality communication.

Your mate, ironically, is probably wrestling with concerns and fears similar to yours. He is, most likely, contending with fears of dying, being disabled, and failing to provide for your family. Even if they don't communicate them, patients confront serious questions: Why do I have heart disease? Why did I survive? Will you still love me? Does this mean I'll die young, without seeing my children grown or my grandchildren born? Communicating these concerns will help both of you confront them.

Surprising realizations, connections, and intimacy can occur only when people communicate. Heart patients, for example, may not realize that their mates have difficulties of their own in a cardiac crisis. One cardiac couple sat in the hospital waiting room while their thirty-eight-year-old son had open-heart surgery. Henry turned to his wife and asked, "Was this how it was for you when you sat waiting during my surgery? I had no idea it was so hard on this side of the knife."

> If it is too difficult to discuss deeper issues, break through the myth of protection by talking about everyday concerns until you're both comfortable talking more intimately.

Decide together if you should take a weekend drive or go to a baseball game, how you can help your children with their college expenses, whether or not you should continue plans to redo the kitchen. Ask your mate where the deed to the house is located, whether he has begun to consider retirement, and so on. Communicating on these topics will pave the way for more intimate conversation.

Myth 2: Stress Is Reduced by Withholding Anger and Other "Negative" Feelings

A popular myth is that if you ignore, repress, or silence anger or other negative feelings, they will go away and stress and discomfort will be successfully avoided. The opposite, however, is true. Feelings exist and persist until felt and released. Stress increases, not decreases, when we suppress our emotions. Sharing them allows us to honestly let go of fear, guilt, and anger.

Communication is strangled by withholding anger and other difficult feelings. These feelings ultimately "come out sideways" in your verbal communication and body language. Honest, respectful expression is replaced with silently clenched fists, bitterness, and barbs. You may even withdraw from communication as an unconscious expression of your repressed feelings.

Dr. Theodore Rubin asserts that expressing anger can actually strengthen relationships.[2] He maintains that expressing anger demonstrates that a mate cares enough to want more intimacy and is willing to invest emotional energy in the relationship. Disclosing your feelings is a statement of confidence that your relationship can withstand difficulties and disagreement.

Make a commitment to start talking openly about your feelings, even the difficult ones. Be generous in your expectations of yourself and your mate. Try to remember that sharing feelings requires courage and trust because doing so makes one vulnerable. The longer it has been since the two of you have disclosed your feelings, the more you will need to ease into sharing them. Begin by taking small steps. The rewards will be a less stressful recovery for both of you and a strengthened relationship.

Myth 3: Good Communication Means Agreement

Wouldn't it be nice if you told your mate that you felt angry and hurt that he hasn't seemed interested in you since he came home from the hospital, and he heard you, agreed with you, and promised to change his behavior? Perhaps. But if you and your spouse agreed about everything, your life together would probably be pretty boring and your relationship unhealthy. It would be hard to determine where you ended and your mate began.

Though it is human nature to avoid conflict, people can and do disagree. Disagreement is a normal and healthy part of relationships. Communicating often highlights differences. But it is only through communication that you and your mate can air, accept, and navigate your differences. Believing that you and your mate should always agree or that your perception is better than his creates tension and distance, putting additional stress on your relationship. It encourages "people pleasing," which leads to a sense of disempowerment and resentment in both of you.

> *Be mindful of what you see.*
> *Always remember,*
> *your focus determines your reality.*[3]

When Ronald's cardiologist recommended open-heart surgery, Ron wanted to schedule it immediately. Tina, in her usual inquisitive style, continued to ask questions and suggested getting a second opinion. She was categorically opposed to him just checking into the hospital. Ron felt anxious and unsupported by Tina. Tina said she couldn't just say yes. She needed more information and time to get used to the idea. Ron refused to consult with another specialist. Tina threatened to wash her hands of it and leave Ron with sole responsibility for the decision. In her anger, she said that if the surgery turned out less than 100 percent, it would be Ron's own fault.

Without the help of a close friend, they might not have been able to mediate their differences. Expressing their fears and their need for each other's love enabled them to appreciate their divergent styles. They reached a decision they both supported.

Good communication requires more than just talking and listening. It is a process of initiating and maintaining respectful interaction with another human being despite your differences. Good communication fosters appreciation and respect of personal differences. It moves you toward empathy, greater understanding, and mutually satisfying solutions to life's challenges.

Personal differences surface during times of illness. Age, gender, family traditions, ethnicity, and cultural heritage also influence how individuals cope with serious illness. It has been thoroughly documented, for example, that Italian, Greek, and Jewish families, which typically engage in intense interactions, are more comfortable explicitly stating their needs during illness. On the other hand, Irish, Scandinavian, and German families, which tend to handle illness with stoic detachment, require support to validate the importance of their needs.[4] It's not that one style is better or worse, easier or more difficult.

> Recognizing the influence of age, gender, family traditions, and ethnicity can help you and your mate understand your differing responses to heart disease.

Knowing how you feel and talk about illness can also help you understand how your mate copes and verbalizes. Acknowledging these differences will make communication easier as you navigate through recovery together.

Hans came home with a certificate honoring him as "Rehab Hero of the Year." Sophia tossed it on a pile of unanswered mail on the kitchen counter. That night she angrily turned from him in bed. When he asked why, she launched into a tirade about how unappreciated she felt. Why, he wouldn't even have attended rehab, she reasoned, if it hadn't been for her effort to get him there so many mornings. Sophia felt hurt and angry, isolated and unrecognized.

Hans expressed his surprise and frustration that she'd "rained on his parade." To him, the award meant that people cared that he was alive and were supportive of his progress. He wanted her to be proud of him, too.

With the help of a counselor, Sophia and Hans are learning how divergent beliefs and feelings can complicate daily living when a chronic illness is a component of their relationship. Both want to find authentic ways to express their love for each other and live in harmony without giving up the truth of their individual experience. Not only is it puzzling for each to understand the other, but they realize that the balance of caring for self and for another person is complex.

Mindfulness—Living in the Moment

Mindfulness, a spiritual concept, can have practical benefits.[5] Practicing mindfulness means using a part of your awareness to focus on experience as you are in it, doing it, living it. It means, simply, learning to pay attention to what you are doing as you do it, rather than focusing on nostalgia for the past or fears about the future. This practice keeps you "in the present moment," the only moment you can experience and control. You will find yourself more alive, energized, and joyful as a result.

> Pay attention to what you are doing while you are doing it. In the present moment you can fully experience yourself and your life.

Knowing what your behaviors, beliefs, motivations, and feelings are *as they are happening* can shift your understanding of who you are. It leads you to an awareness and appreciation of your individuality, your uniqueness. Mindfulness practice is integral to the healing process. As you become more focused on "what makes you tick," you are more likely to accept the uniqueness of others, including your mate, and expect them to have different responses to the same experience.

Mindfulness practice is a foundation from which you can build respectful communication and increase understanding and intimacy. Instead of fearing and resenting your differences, mindfulness can lead each of you to a curiosity about and appreciation of your differing perspectives. You can decide to share what you know about you, and you can invite your mate to share his experience in response. From this curiosity, sharing, and appreciation, you can find solutions that work for both of you.

It may be necessary for you to take the first step toward open and honest communication. Begin with a discrete sharing and assess how it feels. Observe how your invitation to reciprocate is received by your spouse. Don't give up if you're met with a blank stare or a surprised silence. It's worth your effort to try again and again. It can lead to reduced suffering for you, your mate, and the relationship. In time, your mate may follow your lead.

Loving contact and clear communication are more difficult in a time of crisis and when adapting to a chronic illness. Be gentle with yourself and your mate as you engage in improving your communication. Keep your expectations realistic, and celebrate your successes together. Consider the following guidelines as you strive to improve your communication and intimacy.

HEARTMATES®
COMMUNICATION GUIDELINES

Do

Do say how you feel.

Do remember that your
spouse has similar concerns.

Do express your anger.

Do try to understand
your mate's individual
style of expression.

Do respect your own needs.

Do focus on loving each
other.

Do enlist the help of a friend
if you reach an impasse.

Do honor individual
differences.

Don't

Don't withdraw
for fear you'll
stress your mate.

Don't believe the myth
that communication is
harmful.

Don't believe your
relationship is too fragile
to bear your feelings.

Don't be scared off
by differences
between you
and your mate.

Don't forget that
unspoken feelings
"come out sideways."

Don't avoid talking
about important concerns.

Don't forget that
communication
can be difficult.

Don't mistake
disagreement for disapproval.

Sexuality and the Cardiac Relationship

Heartmates of all ages were affected by the sexual revolution of the 1960s. Following publication of the Kinsey Report, a previously taboo subject became a legitimate matter for scientific research and public discussion. Despite that revolution, many people still don't talk easily about their personal sexual activity.

Heart disease causes many cardiac couples to openly explore and discuss sexual issues for the first time. Influenced by parents, teachers, religious authorities, and the media, your values can impair your willingness and ability to talk about sex and sexuality. But propriety and etiquette are less important as you consider what really matters in your life.

> This is a time when both you and your spouse deeply need and strongly fear being connected sexually with each other.

Cardiac recovery provides an opportunity to talk about your sexuality and cultivate sexual expression with your mate.

All cardiac couples have questions about sex. There isn't anyone, regardless of confidence level, who doesn't have some concern about how heart disease will affect their sexual relationship. If you're like most heartmates, for example, you may fear that your sexual relationship has been permanently damaged. (There's no need it should be, as we shall see.) This is an absolutely natural fear, particularly in the beginning stages of recovery. Talk about your fears and concerns with your mate and seek answers to your questions.

It's important to note that, decades after the sexual revolution, it is still rare for medical professionals to initiate a personal discussion or actively solicit a cardiac couple's questions about heart disease and the sexual aspect of their relationship. Though hospital coronary care units often include sex education as part of their overall service to cardiac patients and spouses, sex is so sensitive and personal an issue that it is difficult for most professionals to be completely helpful. You will probably have to take responsibility for asking your questions and demanding answers, as well as seeking alternative resources.

> Take responsibility for initiating the subject of sexual activity with your doctor. Persist until you get the answers and results you seek.

*J*ust *before my husband was released from the hospital after his heart attack, a nurse brought us a tape about sexuality and heart disease. In a flat, mechanical, almost harsh tone, a professional narrator voiced things that were personal and tender for me.*

It made me uncomfortable; it made me angry. I wanted to scream at the voice in the sterile gray machine on the window sill, "How could you understand? I don't care if we ever have intercourse again. I'm terrified that he's going to die." But I said nothing. We laughed together, sort of self-consciously, and turned off the tape. I felt misunderstood and wondered if my concern, or lack of interest in sex, was unusual.

When my husband came home and we were together in our own bed, he put his arms around me and I fell asleep feeling secure and comforted. But weeks passed, and my fears about sex remained overwhelming. I heard echoes from the portable tape recorder, but they didn't diminish my terror. Maybe he would die from the stress or excitement of an orgasm. Or maybe, at forty-three, my sex life as I knew it was over. Perhaps he was impotent, a side effect of his medications. Or maybe he was disinterested, a side effect of heart disease. Maybe I was no longer attractive to him.

Not so liberated that I could ask him directly about what was going on, I kept my fears quiet and they remained unchallenged. I simply was not sure how to broach the subject without humiliating him and embarrassing myself. I know differently now.

There are five major *misconceptions* surrounding the subject of sex and heart disease. Whether consciously or subconsciously, each one of these contributes to feelings of fear, apprehension, unworthiness, and disappointment:

- Sexual activity is hazardous for heart patients.
- Heart disease decreases libido and impairs sexual functioning.
- Heart disease signifies the end of normal sexual activity.
- Sexual prowess is the measure of masculinity, and masculinity is the measure of a man's worth.
- Sex is love.

None of these is true. The remaining material in this chapter will help you replace these misconceptions with more realistic and up-to-date information.

We can start by examining the medical facts about the physical aspects of sexual activity and heart disease. Much of the medical information currently available stems from research with male heart patients, but recent attention to issues of female heart patients promises to yield additional findings soon.[6]

The recommendation to abstain from sex early in recovery may give you the false idea that sexual activity is dangerous for recovering heart patients and that your sexual relationship is over.

> The truth is that the vast majority of patients can and do return to their normal sexual activity within three months of a cardiac event.

The abstinence recommendation is similar to that given to couples who have just had a baby. It is a temporary guideline to allow the patient to rest and recuperate.

It is generally accepted that cardiac patients experience a *temporary* decrease in sexual drive. There are three main reasons for this decline in libido: depression, fatigue, and side effects of medications. These factors usually dissipate over time; if they do not, they can be treated.

In the *Harvard Heart Letter,* Dr. Thomas Hackett, chief of psychiatry at Massachusetts General Hospital and professor of psychiatry at Harvard Medical School, addresses depression, fatigue, and many other questions about sex raised by male heart patients and their mates.[7]

According to Hackett, the depression that commonly follows a heart attack includes reduced feelings of sexual desire. For patients in active recovery, the depression is exacerbated because they are easily fatigued and spend lots of time alone, reflecting on what has happened to them. This depression, a natural response after trauma to the body, diminishes desire. Hackett points out that for 85 percent of patients, the depression and reduced libido pass and never become a major problem.[8] However, if, after three months, depression and reduced sexual interest continue, you should seek the advice of your general practitioner or a mental health professional.

Physically, according to Hackett, "there appears to be no medical basis for implicating satisfying sex, in a familiar and supportive relationship, as a hazard."[9]

> Research done with cardiac couples who had stable, long-term relationships documented that the average amount of energy expended while having sex is equivalent to climbing two flights of stairs.

To reduce your fear about your mate's physical health, watch your mate climb some stairs. Let that information sink in.

Like other physical activity, sexual participation should be resumed gradually during recovery. Dr. Hackett advises that a cardiac couple limit themselves to foreplay and abstain from intercourse for the first two to three weeks of recovery. He makes this suggestion "not because sexual activity is dangerous but because the guideline takes the pressure off both partners to perform." Dr. Hackett continues, stating that "masturbation is also perfectly safe and may ease the transition back to partnered sex. After three weeks there are usually no restrictions, though this schedule may be modified in cases of severe illness."[10]

Frances, a seventy-five-year-old cardiac spouse, recalled a visit with her doctor twenty-five years earlier. Usually reserved and embarrassed, Frances marshaled her courage to ask him about sex. She told her physician that she and her husband had been turning their backs in bed to avoid arousing each other. Both were afraid that sexual activity would endanger his life. Her doctor emphatically informed her that there was no physical risk and that they could safely resume their sexual practice. Frances whispered shyly that it had made their last years together more precious.

In *The Sensuous Heart,* Suzanne Cambre explains the time restrictions for a return to sexual activity. Waiting four to six weeks is recommended for most people after a heart attack. After heart surgery the timing is the same, because it takes about that long for surgical patients to regenerate their strength and for the breastbone to mend. In the absence of a heart attack, patients having an angiogram or angioplasty should wait twenty-four hours for the puncture site to close before returning to physical activity.[11]

The physical position of intercourse appears to make no difference in the amount of stress from sexual activity. There is no medical basis to support one sexual position being safer than another. When the patient is male, many cardiac couples automatically switch to female superior position, thinking that a posture with the male on his back will be less stressful. It is more important that you and your mate choose positions with which you feel confident and comfortable.

Normal body changes that occur during sexual intercourse have nothing to do with heart disease, nor do they endanger a heart patient. Average, middle-aged couples take between ten and sixteen minutes for intercourse. During arousal, skin may flush and breathing, pulse, and blood pressure increase. During orgasm, which lasts less than thirty seconds, the heart works the hardest. The pulse may reach 150 beats a minute, and the blood pressure may exceed 160/90. During resolution, following orgasm, the body returns to its resting rate within a matter of seconds.

It is true that some heart patients experience palpitations or angina during intercourse.

> Angina should not mean the end of sexual activity.
> For the minority of people who experience angina
> during intercourse, doctors can prescribe medica-
> tions that can be taken before sex.

These drugs can help prevent chest discomfort.[12] Call your doctor and ask about these medications if discomfort lasts longer than fifteen minutes. Angina should not mean the end of sexual activity.

Some medications used to lower blood pressure, prevent palpitations, or control angina may, as a side effect, diminish libido or produce impotence. Prescription drugs also may have the effect of reducing natural lubrication in female cardiac patients. Work with your doctor to find medications that don't have these side effects.

For some heart patients, impotence or diminished libido can persist even after medications have been adjusted. This could indicate a physical condition, which can be treated. The American Heart Association's 2001 pamphlet *Sex and Heart Disease* addresses a new drug used to treat male impotence and the potential benefits and risks it has for heart patients.[13] Get your cardiologist's advice about use of this medication. Persisting impotence or diminished libido can also be an indication of unresolved depression. Consult your primary doctor or a mental health professional if your symptoms continue for more than three months.

Although it is normal to feel apprehensive about resuming sexual activity, and there may be some changes to the way you express yourselves sexually after a cardiac event, most couples make an adjustment. Open communication and a willingness to consult your doctor if you have prolonged difficulties is key. And perhaps the best thing is that you will come to appreciate the physical closeness more and celebrate your return to sexual activity as a deepening of your intimacy and love.

Sexuality and Self-Image

Heart disease challenges the self-image of both patient and heartmate, including body image and our view of ourselves as sexual beings.

Confronting these aspects of who we really are is part of the work of reclaiming or developing a healthy sexual intimacy with our partners. Both men and women still have difficulty accepting their bodies and their sexuality.

Hospitalized heart patients fear they are dying. Their real concerns about sexuality only begin once they feel confident about surviving. Patients who flirt with nurses are most likely experiencing shock and denial. Nurses frequently misinterpret this bravado and fail to understand the denial, fear, and insecurity resting just below the surface.

Recovering male heart patients, coping with a changing self-image, naturally question their virility. The notion that masculinity is measured by sexual prowess sorely needs revision. This misconception affects male cardiac patients of all ages, adding unnecessary pressure to their physical and emotional recovery.

Recovering female patients, adapting to a changing self-image, naturally question whether they will still be sexually attractive to their partner. The notion that femininity is measured by bodily perfection and beauty needs to be changed as well. The fear that a woman's attractiveness is lost because of a "disfiguring" scar reduces self-worth.

Some cardiac couples return to normal sexual activity as though nothing has happened. Sex, used as proof that everything's fine, is only a temporary cover-up. It's confusing, when both of you know that things aren't fine or "just as they used to be," to pretend that everything is the same. A frank discussion of sex can heal that agonizing pretense.

Cardiac patients may jokingly refer to themselves as "damaged goods." This may reflect a fear of impotence, of being unable to perform like a "whole" person. You may hesitate to encourage your mate to return to sexual activity for fear of intensifying feelings of inadequacy. But avoiding intimacy will only aggravate the problem. Joking may distract you both from taking that first difficult step toward a healthy sexual relationship: discussing the situation seriously.

As a heartmate, you, too, may be forced to cope with a changing self-image that affects your sexuality. A full year into recovery, one forty-nine-year-old heartmate acknowledged that she couldn't bring herself to be sexual very often. Although she didn't entirely understand why, she carried around an uneasy feeling that both she and her husband had suddenly gone from being young and attractive to being "over the hill." Another heartmate beautifully expressed how heart disease had been an opportunity for her to change her body image: "I was never very satisfied with my body as a young woman. Now, in my fifties, a heartmate, I'm just discovering that my body is a source of pleasure and comfort."

> Heart disease can be an opportunity to revise your body image and accept yourself as a sexual person.

Recovery may temporarily inhibit your sex life. But heart disease may not be the only factor to consider. Whether or not you have noticed, the frequency and style of your sexual relationship has changed gradually over the years. Some natural decline in frequency of intercourse is documented in people over the age of forty. Heart disease may accelerate that change or bring the natural decline into focus.

It's unrealistic to try to maintain a standard that was established in your twenties and thirties. Television suggests that youth, power, and success are what counts, contributing to the pressure to perform. But maturity and comfort are equally valuable. Over time you can accept your mate's habit of nodding off during the late night news. Let's face it, you're probably not so focused, witty, or romantic late at night, either. But you can enjoy, appreciate, even relish the softer, quieter, and more vulnerable ways you are sexual with each other.

With the onset of heart disease, some couples have sexual concerns they never had before, although these are commonly related to feelings and images, not to physical changes or dangers. The cause does not make the concern any less real. For some couples the problem stems from their interpretation of physical limitations; for others, it's their outdated body images and unexamined attitudes about sexual attractiveness (in other words, shame or fear of being rejected); for still others, there's the fear of endangering the patient's health or life.

Solutions may be found in talking, trusting, and trying out behaviors together. Go slowly! Don't be pushed by external forces that suggest it's time to "go back to normal." But don't let helplessness or hopelessness win the day, either. Together, the two of you can find the right balance.

Beyond Facts about Sexuality

Facts and information can help facilitate greater intimacy and a return to a satisfying sexual relationship, but they're no substitute for communication.

> Be honest about your need for intimacy. Here, as in other areas of your relationship, you will find that you and your mate differ, sometimes significantly and other times in minor ways.

One of you may be eager to resume a sexual relationship, while the other may be more reticent. Be patient and kind with each other. Each of you has expectations and fears that need to be aired, respected, and worked through.

You are separate individuals *and* you are allies, members of the same team. Being teammates is especially essential when it comes to something as sensitive and personal as sex. Heart disease provides the opportunity to examine your changing sexual intimacy in a way that gradual aging doesn't. It offers a chance to see each other with new eyes and to discover a new appreciation of one another.

Both of you need to give and receive physical intimacy and comfort. Most couples are able eventually to return to precrisis sexual activity. In the great majority of cases, there is no medical contraindication to doing so. As time passes, however, changes in your mate's physical health may require further adjustments. It will be up to you to face and make these adjustments together.

If the severity of your mate's heart disease results in you being unable to have intercourse, it is a real loss, one you can grieve and resolve together. Avoid the temptation to deny your needs. Denying the need for physical intimacy, avoiding the pain of talking about it, reduces your opportunity of discovering new ways to be with each other sexually. Together, you and your mate can muster the effort, courage, and creativity to face what you have lost and to find new ways to express your caring physically.

Many cardiac couples find themselves closer after the cardiac crisis than during any other period in their relationship. The cardiac experience may have changed your values and priorities. Petty irritations and aggravating differences seem unimportant in light of the bond that heart disease has threatened. You may feel freer to be openly appreciative of your mate's affection, more direct about your needs, and more willing to give. The threat of loss may ultimately open your hearts to each other.

Regardless of how close they may be, it isn't unusual for cardiac couples to confront an emotional barrier to intimacy consisting of unexpressed fear, resentment, or anger. Some heartmates hold back, distrustful about depending on their mates and fearful of disappointment. It's hard to make love before these feelings are released and forgiven.

Perhaps one of the most significant distinctions to clarify is that *sex is not love,* although it is often mistaken for it. Whether your sexual expression includes or precludes sexual intercourse, what's important is that you and your mate find a way to express your love. As one heartmate stated, "Of course, sex is only the frosting on the cake—but how I love frosting." No matter the level and style of your sexual activity, recognize that it can be more than sport, pleasure, or comfort. Sexual expression can be one way to fully experience yourself and connect with your partner. Sex has been described as the momentary miracle of transcending time and space. Perhaps the most distorted and violated of our expressions, sex is potentially a sacred and beautiful spiritual and physical act.

Cardiac couples can adapt to changes in sexual expression more easily if they have faith in the love that bonds them. And there are so many ways to express love: a touch, a kiss, a caress, and sexual intercourse are a few examples of the rich repertoire human beings have to express themselves. Scheduling time together is a way to say that your relationship has a special priority in your lives. Make a date to give or get a back rub, to cuddle, or to make love. Saying "I love you" goes a long way, too. If you maintain open hearts and open minds, you will discover expressions of love that are right for you.

> Once you've opened up about your feelings, talk about your differences respectfully and lovingly. Discuss resolutions that take both your needs into account.

Communication doesn't solve all problems, but conflicts and unmet needs hidden in the back of your mind can grow out of proportion. Ask each other for what you want and need. Your intimate communication can relieve the anguish of unmet sexual expectations and performance anxiety while strengthening your love bond. It can lead to physical intimacy that is mutually satisfying.

Strive to open your hearts to one another, to share your feelings and concerns. Remember, too, that with or without heart disease, none of us knows how long we have to live a satisfying life. If you express your love today and you find yourself together tomorrow, you are blessed with more precious time to live and love.

As you heal your relationship together, give sexual activity its appropriate value in your life. Do not under- or overestimate its worth. Your connection to each other needs revitalization and support in order to heal. Your sexual relationship is a symbol of your love and your union. It is a way to celebrate life and your bond as heartmates.

Healing the Heartmate Relationship

Constructive and creative change requires the willingness to examine your relationship, the vulnerability to hope for increased intimacy, the trust and compassion to forgive each other for past disappointments, and the persistence to plan and carry out small, everyday adjustments. Renew your commitment to your relationship.

Before we continue our discussion on healing relationships, it's important to acknowledge that, sadly, there are those for whom the cardiac crisis is the event that precipitates a final break in the relationship. Cindy, a forty-seven-year-old cardiac spouse, described that she and her fifty-two-year-old husband, Dick, were considering a legal separation when he suffered a heart attack. Months of recovery passed. Dick's response to his disease was irritability, and he directed his anger at Cindy. There was no more discussion about a separation.

Her dilemma was a catch-22. It had been complicated, for all the usual reasons, to consider divorce. She had struggled with the difficult questions: Could she create a new life for herself? Where would she find support when most of her family and friends were married and loyal to them as a couple? Their marriage was no longer right. But now, with Dick's heart attack, Cindy was afraid of being cast as a selfish, insensitive, irresponsible woman, turning her back on a sick man like a captain abandoning a sinking ship.

No one would advise a couple to separate or divorce during recovery because of the additional stress. Yet there are relationships that cannot be healed. Eroded trust is difficult for couples to rebuild in any situation. The cardiac event, a betrayal by the body, may be experienced as a further abandonment. In these cases, one or both partners have usually given up hope and are unwilling to put any more effort and goodwill into the relationship. If this is your situation, accept your partner's limits, and stay or go based on your own.[14] It is wise to seek professional help to provide both of you the support and guidance you need to work through this major life change.

> One of the most important elements of healing any relationship is rebuilding the trust that was threatened or shattered.

All human beings live with the fundamental fear of being abandoned. Heartmates react to this threat in a variety of ways, from being overly protective to feigning fierce independence. Acknowledge your fear of being left, first to yourself and then to your mate, as a prerequisite for healing the trust between you. Your spouse can't realistically guarantee that he'll be there for you . . . forever. That is difficult and painful to admit.

> Once you can accept that there is no guarantee of forever, you can begin anew, planning for a future that includes an appreciation of the ephemeral, uncertain nature of life.

Whatever the state of your relationship, your challenge is to see the reality and make peace with it. Only then is there the opportunity to take advantage of a new perspective, to reconnect based on mutual appreciation and respect. Your marriage bond may be strengthened by surviving this experience together.

As serious and significant as your relationship is, nothing is a more powerful healer than humor. Being able to laugh at yourselves and your situation will help you see things as they truly are and enjoy your togetherness. The great comedian, Victor Borge, said that laughter was the shortest distance between two people.

Anne reported that funny movies helped them pass many hours during Mark's recovery from open-heart surgery. More significantly, the films gave them something to enjoy together. Mark complained of pain when he aggravated his incision by laughing too hard, but they were both able to find humor even in this. Laughter is healing.

Finally, repairing the heartmate connection depends on how well the balance between the individuals' needs and the relationship's needs can be negotiated. A healthy relationship requires each partner to establish and protect individuality and simultaneously reach out to care about each other. This is right responsibility and healthy interdependence. "A good marriage is one in which each appoints the other guardian of his solitude."[15] This is a complex challenge that promises great rewards.

Once the realization is accepted
that even between the closest human beings
infinite distances continue to exist,
a wonderful living side by side can grow up,
if they succeed in loving the distance between them,
which makes it possible for each to see the other
whole against the sky.[16]

SUGGESTIONS FOR HEALING
YOUR HEARTMATE CONNECTION

• Share your feelings with each other.
• Cherish your time together.
• Give yourself permission to be romantic.
• Experiment with new ways to express your love.
• Make realistic plans for your future.
• Mark anniversaries of recovery.
• Let yourselves laugh and have fun.
• Celebrate being alive and together.

Chapter 8 Notes

1. Edward J. Speedling, *Heart Attack: The Family Response at Home and in the Hospital* (New York: Tavistock Publications, 1982), 162.
2. Theodore Isaac Rubin, MD, *The Angry Book* (New York: Macmillan, 1969), 168–69.
3. Wisdom from the Jedi master, Qui-Gon Jinn, to young Anakin Skywalker in *Star Wars: Episode One: The Phantom Menace*, George Lucas, dir. (Lucasfilm/Twentieth Century Fox, 2000).
4. Monica McGoldrick, *Ethnicity and Family Therapy* (New York: Guilford Press, 1996). McGoldrick's groundbreaking work is full of wisdom and

heart. It continues to assist family therapists and healthcare professionals in their work with families of diverse backgrounds.

5. Studies by Jon Kabat-Zinn and his colleagues have demonstrated that bringing a fullness of attention to whatever is occurring in the here and now fosters the healing process. See "Commentary—Daily Experiences of Relationships and Illness: Reflecting on Our Focus," George William Saba, PhD, in *Families, Systems & Health*, vol. 17, no. 3 (1999): 291; and "Couples' Experience of Illness: The Daily Lives of Patients and Spouses," David W. Young, MA, and David Rosenthal, PhD, in *Families, Systems & Health*, vol. 17, no. 3 (1999): 265–85.

6. I direct you to an important organization, WomenHeart. This organization will be useful to female heart patients and their mates, providing up-to-date information on heart disease in women. Visit the WomenHeart Web site at <www.womenheart.org>.

7. Thomas Hackett, MD, "Men and Sex after a Heart Attack," *Harvard Heart Letter*, vol. 11, no. 5 (March 1986): 5–6.

8. More recent studies published in professional journals indicate that a much larger percent of heart patients experience a lasting depression.

9. Hackett, 6. A Japanese study analyzing the cause of 5,000 sudden deaths found that of the victims, thirty-four died (presumably) during intercourse. Of those, thirty were with partners other than their own spouses. Virtually all had blood levels close to, or in the range of, intoxication. These data suggest that the lethal stress was not caused by intercourse, but by intercourse in combination with alcohol and in the context of an extramarital affair.

10. Ibid., 6.

11. Suzanne Cambre, RN, BSHA, *The Sensuous Heart* (Atlanta: Pritchett & Hull Associates, 1978).

12. Cambre, 13, 19.

13. The 2001 revised edition of *Sex and Heart Disease,* published by the American Heart Association. Call for a copy at (800) 242-8721.

14. Stephen C. Paul, *Inneractions: Visions to Bring Your Inner and Outer Worlds into Harmony* (San Francisco: Harper, 1992).

15. Rainer Maria Rilke, *Letters of Rainer Maria Rilke, 1910–1926* (New York: W. W. Norton, 1969).

16. Ibid.

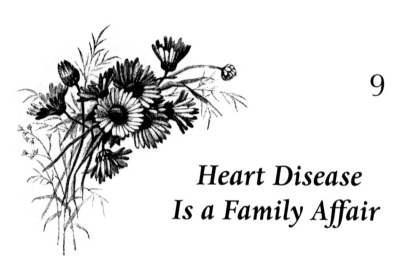

Heart Disease Is a Family Affair

Life with heart disease is truly a family affair. The unexpected and life-threatening onset of heart disease ruptures the fabric of the family, which cries out to be healed. When one member of the family is wounded, every member is indelibly scarred. The effects on the family's unity may last a lifetime. Effects differ depending on the patient's familial role, the timing of the illness in the family life cycle, and the openness of the family system. Uncertainty and unpredictability replace expectations of safety and security.

> Heart disease can also provide families an opportunity. Inherent within the crisis is the potential for increased understanding, intimacy, nurturing, and support.

Family members, temporarily more vulnerable and sensitive, may drop defenses, forgive old hurts, and reach out to each other with caring and love.

Heart Disease and Family Diversity

Waiting during open-heart surgery was excruciating. Our thirteen-year-old daughter, Debbie, chose to be at the hospital with me rather than go to school. We sat together surrounded by friends.

By midmorning I felt restless and asked Debbie to go for a walk with me. We made our way, holding hands, to a single-treed island in the urban hospital block and stood together under the sun.

I suggested that we do a visualization for her dad. We imagined the warmth and radiance of the sun entering the operating room, strengthening the surgical staff, and filling the surgical suite with healing light. We visualized energy and prayers coming from our friends all over the country. We saw ourselves as channels, allowing energy to flow through us and into the hospital to her dad and his surgical team.

I felt especially blessed to have a child who would share such a prayer with me. Later we decided we needed another walk, so we returned to our island. With traffic whizzing by, we closed our eyes and held hands again. This time Debbie led our personal meditation.

When the chaplain brought the news that "the repair had been successful and they were closing," Debbie and I held each other, our tears of joy and gratitude mingling. Suddenly we were starving, and we celebrated with a late lunch.

It is ideal when family members can support each other in a crisis. Unfortunately this doesn't always happen. A family crisis can offer an opportunity to heal old rifts and resentments, but it can also intensify conflicts and magnify misunderstandings. The family has the basic strength and resilience of any institution that maintains itself over generations. But within all families there are painful scars and unhealed wounds.

The acute crisis automatically makes the spouse the anchor of the family. You become solely responsible for your children: their activities, school, appointments, meals, and other arrangements. If your children are older, already launched, you become the director of communications, sharing the good and bad news with them. Family members often revert to earlier roles and behaviors. Your grown children may feel as needy and dependent on you as when they were toddlers. It can fall on you to respond to everyone's emotional needs.

The stress of being the family mainstay may not at first be obvious. But consider the weight you're carrying on your shoulders. If you're like most cardiac spouses, you're preoccupied with your mate's recovery, and you're worried about how upset your children are. You may be concerned about where the next paycheck will come from, how next month's bills will be paid, and the last thing you want is for your children to know you're worried. You're distressed about leaving your mate's side and, simultaneously, feel guilty about not giving other members of your family enough time and attention.

Being the family's anchor makes you aware of how powerfully your spouse's illness affects all family members. It does *not* mean that you can attend to or fix every problem or that you're responsible for healing unpleasant or painful relationships in the family. Responsible leadership means accepting and respecting family members' needs as they, too, progress through this unknown terrain.

> Your primary responsibility to your children is to inform them about what has happened and to keep them updated. If you have young children, you have the added responsibility of caring for them.

Common sense should guide your decision making when it comes to communicating facts about what has happened. Gauge what information is appropriate for your younger children. Resist the temptation, however, to keep secrets from them. Adult children should be informed as soon as possible. But even this rule has its exceptions.

Dana worried that her daughter Michelle would have a miscarriage after learning that her dad had experienced a heart attack. Michelle lived hundreds of miles away and was in the eighth month of a difficult pregnancy. Dana weighed the possible consequences of informing Michelle or withholding the information. She tried to take all factors into consideration: the severity of his condition, which was still medically unclear, Michelle's need to see her father, his need to be comforted by his daughter, and the new baby's safe arrival.

School and other social institutions pay little or no attention to the needs of the children of heart patients, although they often provide help for selected stress experiences such as divorce or the death of a parent. Unless children openly express their feelings, most adults will not be aware of what they are going through. Heart patients themselves are routinely surprised when their children tell them how deeply the illness has affected them.

In most cases, children's feelings and concerns are ignored or swept aside, either because of our ignorance (not realizing that they are equally affected by a family member's heart disease) or because our own concerns are so consuming. Cardiackids are expected to be fine because their parent is recovering. If the family shrouds the heart disease in secrecy, children may not even know that a parent is ill.

Families can be tortured by secrets demanded by the heart patient.[1] Some patients use secrets to avoid deep fear and shame. It's not uncommon for a patient to impose silence on the family because of concerns about job security or of not being promoted because of heart disease. Sometimes fear and shame will manifest as superstition: If we don't talk about it, the problem will go away and nothing worse will happen. What they don't realize is that secrets actually complicate recovery and can harm their families.

A successful executive was airlifted from a mountain ski resort to a hospital cardiac care unit in the nearest major city. All four grown children and his grandchildren witnessed the event. Each was astounded, shocked, horrified—and silenced. The executive forbade them to mention what had happened.

One daughter, who lived across the country, grieved deeply. Terrified that she'd never be able to tell her father how much she loved him, she berated her mother long distance. "Talk to him, make him understand, persuade him to release all of us from this vow of silence." The heartmate, paralyzed and torn between her two loves, her husband and her children, felt powerless and despairing.

Another heart patient released his family from the secret only after he had a cardiac arrest in public, on a municipal softball field. A year of hiding the truth, maintaining the pretense of no heart disease, had strangled the family's interaction and halted their mourning and recovery.

> Having to keep heart disease a secret is torture for
> the family. In order to heal, cardiackids need to talk
> about the powerful impressions and images that
> haunt their dreams and waking hours.

Cardiackids have feelings they need to understand and express. They
experience the fear of nearly being left without a parent, the guilt of
believing they caused the cardiac event, and the shock of their secure
world becoming permanently uncertain. Demanding secrecy or consciously practicing silence makes healing impossible. If you can't
change the situation within the family, it is imperative that you access
a respected adult (such as an extended family member, teacher, coach,
mentor, religious leader, or professional counselor) who will listen to
the concerns of your children. If no one is available on a regular basis,
encourage your children to write their feelings in a journal.

Roles and Rules

As the heartmate, you are the liaison for all other family members.
Regardless of your relationship with them, they each have genuine
feelings toward your mate and a real stake in his recovery. Relatives
with whom you normally have minimal contact may be more visible
than usual. Depending on how your family gets along, association
with relatives can be a blessing or a burden. This complicates your role
as liaison. You need to set rules and guidelines to care for and protect
yourself and your mate, while simultaneously considering the needs
of other family members.

Virginia, a forty-one-year-old cardiac spouse, had difficulty
keeping Lyle's family's visits to a minimum. She was worried that he
wouldn't tell them when he was too exhausted for visitors. Although
the youngest in her own family, Virginia could be efficient and
tough. She established two periods during the day when guests
could come. When the visiting period was over, she personally ush-
ered everyone out.

One morning, after being told that Lyle was napping and couldn't be disturbed, his oldest sister asked to see Virginia's police badge. The sister informed her, in a condescending tone, that the family didn't appreciate being told when and for how long they could visit their own brother.

It had been three weeks since Lyle's heart attack, so Virginia relaxed the rules. She was surprised when Lyle asked her to reinstate them, expressing appreciation that she had protected him. He still tired easily and found it uncomfortable to ask guests to leave.

Making decisions that take everyone's needs into account is practically impossible. Try to be sensitive; prepare yourself with the understanding that it's inevitable for your priorities to clash with others'. And remember, your first responsibility is to yourself and your recovering mate.

Barbara, a devoted wife, complained that her mother-in-law was sabotaging the heart-healthy diet she had instituted since Arnold's angioplasty procedure. Twice a week, every week, Mildred continued to deliver the home-cooked treats that she had always made to please her son. Butter-laden pastries and salty soups were her specialties. And her cooking was delicious!

Barbara understood that preparing food offered a way for Mildred to express her love for her son, but she knew she had to put her foot down. "Either heart-healthy recipes or no recipes," Barbara finally told Mildred. The new dietary rules included Mildred, and there would be no exceptions.

In a family crisis, it sometimes feels as if there are too many cooks in the kitchen. Usually passive relatives may suddenly become opinionated and expressive when the health of one of their own is at stake. Decision making gets complicated when affected family members differ as to appropriate actions.

> Be open to hearing others' opinions. At the same time, remember that you and your mate are responsible for your recovery.

You are the final arbiter of these decisions. As heartmate, the buck stops with you. This demands both your assertiveness and a willingness to carefully weigh differing opinions.

Jon, a rather shy and taciturn man, described his dilemma after his wife of eighteen years had a heart attack. Her family, large and vociferous, met every evening to hash over the pros and cons of Lois' treatment. When the cardiologist advised open-heart surgery, Lois' family convened in earnest. Jon felt left out and powerless as they argued back and forth late into the night. They finally agreed on the "right" course of action, informing Jon that he should tell the doctor of their decision. At no point was his opinion solicited.

If you honestly believe that other family members are interfering with your mate's recovery, do whatever is needed to protect yourself and your spouse. A word of caution: it is easy to use a family crisis to lay blame or vent past bitterness. Playing the cop—for example, monitoring visiting hours or excluding close relatives from decision making—may mask an unconscious desire to use your power and authority to hurt others.

Family members act according to existing behavior patterns that repeat themselves for generations. Each individual has unique roles in his or her family. When a family crisis hits, everyone automatically reverts to the familiar, well-established roles. Sometimes these work well in helping the family cope, but old, habitual roles can snarl an already complicated situation.

A thirty-six-year-old cardiackid explained how she and her sister assumed their typical roles during their mother's hospitalization. One sister was in charge of cosmetic concerns; the other handled the emotional issues. To keep her mother's spirits up, the former shopped for a new robe and nightgowns for their mother; she made sure her mom's makeup was fresh and her hair coifed. The latter translated the doctors' reports and facilitated communication among the three generations of the family.

> All family members are needed during a crisis. Each member of your family is an individual with unique

> gifts. Appreciating each other's contributions is an
> essential part of pulling together.

If one member of your family is best at interpreting medical information, he or she should handle that. If another has always been the clown, humor has its place, too. All family members, simply by virtue of their love and concern, have a legitimate and valuable role in the process of recovery.

Concerns Cardiackids Confront

The effects of the cardiac crisis on family members may not be readily apparent. On the surface, your family might seem the same as usual. But it's not the same. Adults and children alike, whether well or ill, deal with sudden change by becoming self-absorbed in their feelings and behaviors. Until this passes, family members can't fully participate in healing the family by reopening communication and rebuilding trust. The long, cold fingers of uncertainty touch every family member. With the loss of certainty comes the urge to control and the yearning for order in a world suddenly strange, frightening, and uncontrollable.

> The basic human fear of being abandoned, of being
> left helpless and alone, is both an immediate and
> long-range concern for cardiackids of all ages.

If you are a parent, you are no doubt worried about the effects on your children. Since the onset of heart disease may occur in young, middle-aged, or older people, the needs of children differ from family to family. Within your family, each of your children will have individual needs depending on age, personality, role relationships, and familial responsibilities.

Your children's reactions to the cardiac crisis can vary. They may exaggerate their normal behavior or display unusual behavior that is difficult to understand. Young children may act out their fears through play. You may notice your seven-year-old, for example, play doctor or ambulance driver, which may be her way of making order of the chaos. Children may react unconsciously with physical ailments or symptoms. One heartmate described her shock when she was called by the middle school nurse. Her son had gone to the nurse's office with chest pains, sure that he was having a heart attack.

Your ten-year-old may refuse to play with friends, suddenly becoming solicitous and parental, sensing your fatigue and vulnerability, reversing the normal roles of parent and child. Your adolescent son, struggling to achieve manhood and fearful about losing his father, may take over and try to be "the man of the house."

Your adult children will probably respond in differing ways, too. Children involved in the family business, for example, may find decision making difficult when the authority figure is suddenly unavailable for counsel. Your independent, single daughter, usually too busy to talk, might start dropping by every evening after work, disregarding her personal routine and social life. Grown children might also revert to earlier family roles, feeling insecure as leaders at work or as parents in their own family.

> Cardiac spouses normally try to appear strong and competent so that their children will feel safe. Ironically, cardiackids often interpret this strong, silent facade as: "Don't ask! Don't talk about it." And they don't.

Attuned to your stress level, your children may try to cope with their own stress by guarding their feelings closely. The only way your children may know to be cooperative and helpful is by not demanding your attention, not rocking the boat, or by trying to meet your needs instead of attending to their own.

Unexpressed feelings can fester and leave permanent scars. Once cardiackids are shaken by the knowledge that their parents are mortal, they will never again be innocent. The illusion of security is forever broken.

Edward, now fifty-eight, was ten years old when his father suffered a heart attack. Whenever he and his brother made the least bit of noise, their mother would come out of the kitchen or bedroom looking frightened and say, "Shhh . . . shhh." Edward was terrified that any noise he made would kill his father. He became more and more withdrawn.

Recalling those days, Edward remembered that his family never talked about his father's illness or what was happening to them. One evening at the supper table his terror surfaced. His question echoed through the kitchen: "Will Daddy die?" His mother pushed her chair away from the table and ran crying into the bathroom. The rest of the family finished supper in silence.

After almost fifty years, Edward's memories are still vivid. The trauma of having been a cardiackid returned when his wife, Florence, had a heart attack. Once he shared his memories and feelings, he was able to cope with the present. Florence's heart attack was an opportunity for Edward to heal an old wound.

This excerpt from Interactive Connections, a page on the Heartmates Web site <www.heartmates.com>, poignantly expresses the concerns of a grieving adult daughter as she tries to manage her complex and often conflicting feelings about her mother and her mother's heart disease:

> *The bypass came after her second heart attack. My mom has so much more life to live, and some days she acknowledges this. Other days, she feels so lousy that she is angry, hostile, and depressed.*
>
> *I do not recall her being an especially doting mother when I was a child, and she and I have not been close in my adult years. She has kept me at arm's length despite my desire to know her, and I'm just not sure why.*
>
> *To add to this, I now live 600 miles from her and have a toddler to care for. Each hospitalization is like a nightmare, and I need to grapple with the inevitable truth of her mortality and decide if I need to get up there.*
>
> *I was there for her surgery and again when her congestive heart failure took a turn for the worse. I feel some assurance in that my*

*brother lives in her town and is there for her daily, but I struggle daily
with my feelings of helplessness, anger, sadness, and frustration. I
have a pretty good understanding of her medical treatment, and her
cardiologist is a most wonderful communicator.*

*So I guess I'm writing to find out if there is anyone else out there
dealing with unresolved end-of-life issues with a loved parent who
has heart disease.*

This daughter's account mirrors the universal concerns of adult cardiackids. We struggle to manage our grief about the impending loss of a parent while trying to balance our own adult lives, full with responsibilities for our own families. As we reflect on our lifelong relationship with our sick parent, we feel our disappointment for what might have been. Our idealized images and dreams are exposed as we face the reality of the relationship as it is, often a complicated mixture of imperfect communication, regrets, and lost opportunities for intimacy.

> Heart disease can be an opportunity for cardiac
> families to make a new beginning. We have time to
> grieve, to reflect on and express the complex
> family relationships, to understand our family's
> patterns from a fresh perspective.

There is the possibility for healing. Hope, realistic optimism, and courage meet, providing a new opportunity to heal and love across the generations.

Role Reversals

Changes in family relationships occur as a result of one member's serious illness. Heart disease can mark the beginning of the role reversal that comes with aging. If the onset of heart disease means that the patient does not return to work, for example, adult children may begin to help parents financially. Parents, used to being in charge, have to adjust to being progressively more dependent on their children. And children, used to being cared for, are confronted with the difficulty of assuming more responsibility and caregiving. This role reversal can be especially upsetting, difficult, and heartbreaking for young children.

Rosalee was concerned for her twelve-year-old son. Ever since Rob's dad suffered a heart attack, Rob had assumed responsibility for all the physical work around the house. Snow-shoveling is a major undertaking in their northern winter.

On the surface, such a change in family responsibility seems simple and uncomplicated. But each winter, tensions rose in the family. Rob's dad was ashamed that he was physically unable to shovel and had to leave the entire job to Rob. He paced from window to window, scrutinizing Rob, watching every flake he moved. Rob shoveled, proud of the job he was doing and hoping he would hear praise from his dad.

When Rob finished and entered the house, his father, unable to express his guilt, either criticized the quality of Rob's work or commented on how he ought to have done it. The scene usually ended with Rob slamming the door to his room and isolating himself for the rest of the day. And since each year brought new snow, winter continued to be a stormy time, symbolizing the difficult role changes that heart disease had brought their family.

Less dramatic but just as painful are changes that occur as aging parents become more dependent on grown children who are busy with their own families and careers. Sunday dinners and holiday celebrations, long the pride of the parents, are assumed by the next generation. Children may need to arrange for their parents' doctor visits, transport them when they can no longer drive, and take charge of their outings.

Children may take over these tasks lovingly or grudgingly, and parents may give them up graciously or stubbornly. All of these changes can be difficult to face and accept. Professional family counseling may improve coping and communication skills. It may be helpful to consider, too, that these role reversals can offer a great gift.

> Role reversals provide an opportunity for parents
> and grown children to spend more intimate time
> together, enjoying each other, remembering the
> past, talking, just being together.

Many middle-aged cardiac couples find it a difficult adjustment to accept help, especially from their children. For most of us, giving is easier than receiving. Many of us are accustomed to the role of caregiver or protector and are unpracticed and awkward in the art of receiving. Others may feel undeserving or unworthy of gifts.

You and your mate may find yourselves sandwiched between your grown children and your aging parents. When heart disease complicates the already difficult demands of being part of the "sandwich generation," you may be chronically exhausted and literally overwhelmed.

> You may conclude that you aren't able to do it all.
> And you'd probably be right. Choose where to put
> your energy.

Accustomed and efficient as you may be in the role of caregiver, the additional energy required to deal with heart disease may make you unable to give much to your children or your parents. And neither the young nor the aged may be prepared or able to give you the care you need right now.

> You cannot do it all yourself. Don't be reluctant to
> solicit help from family and friends. Reach out to all
> available resources for help.

Many people will welcome the opportunity to contribute to your recovery process, including members of your extended family. And your immediate family can give, too. Even young children can make worthy contributions and find comfort in being needed. (Make sure to assess that what you're asking of them is age-appropriate and doable—right responsibility—and to thank them.) Other sources of help are available through local social service agencies. The social worker at your hospital may be able to connect you with an appropriate agency. Your church or synagogue may also provide resources to assist you. If you have the financial means, you might consider professional assistance (such as a cleaning service, a childcare service, or a home healthcare service).

Dealing with Cardiackids

Your love for your children makes you naturally concerned about their reaction to the cardiac crisis. Perhaps you feel that you must be more in charge than usual in order to compensate for their feelings of insecurity. You are the one who assumes the role of intermediary between your children and your sick spouse, keeping each filled in on how the other is doing during hospitalization.

You might relay messages and deliver photos of the children or special cards or drawings they've made to lift his spirits. But nothing is as satisfying as direct contact between children and their parent. As soon as your mate is moved from intensive care to a recovery unit, inquire about visits. If young children are restricted from visiting, you can arrange daily phone communication between your mate and the kids. Calls need not be long, but it is affirming and encouraging for them to hear his voice. Sharing a good-night kiss over the phone is better than nothing at all.

Over the long term, you need to detach from negotiating family relationships. Trying to maintain or improve others' relationships doesn't work. You may be tempted to step in and help when you see your spouse and your adult children struggling to establish communication. They may have conflicts to resolve, new things to talk about, or love to express to each other. If there is stress or enmity between your mate and your children, a health crisis may ignite it. You face the impossible paradox: maintaining your alliance with your mate while simultaneously protecting your children.

> Engage in your relationships with your mate and
> your children, but give them the space they need
> to work out their own relationships without your
> interference.

Reassured by a parent's safe return from the hospital, children may begin to express feelings of fear or anger over what they experienced as abandonment and neglect. Less able to speak directly about what's bothering them, younger children's reactions may take the form of poor school performance, depression, an inability to get along with siblings, or accident-prone behavior.

Juggling your needs for privacy and support with your children's increased demands is a tricky balancing act. You want to be there for them at a time when it takes all your energy just to take care of yourself and your mate.

The impulse to protect your children from pain and anguish is universal. But the truth is that it's impossible to do. The cardiac event has occurred. You, your mate, *and* your children have been and will continue to be affected. Even if you could protect your children from reality, it wouldn't necessarily be doing them a favor. Learning to cope with crisis and to accept the realities of life, including illness, is a valuable part of growing up.

There is no such thing as a perfect parent. The pressure of being a heartmate makes parenting even more challenging. If you're not as patient and responsive as usual, keep in mind that you have been parenting alone, without your main source of support, your mate.

A good rule of thumb in dealing with children of any age is to remember that kids are people, too. In a health crisis, children have questions and they have feelings. A child, no matter what age, has the right to be informed about what is happening to his or her parent and family. Take time to listen to and answer children's questions. Let them know how you're feeling and why you may be less patient and available. Children respond well to respect and honesty.

Your Children's Right to Know

Children, even adult children, don't have the same access to hospital staff as you do. They aren't around as much, and hospital staff may not take the time to respond to their questions seriously. Hospital regulations might prohibit young children from visiting at all.

Nothing is more fearful than the unknown. Even though you may not understand the details of every conversation you have with the medical staff, you do experience some relief from being given regular progress reports and information. Your children may not understand every detail either, and they, too, will feel reassured if you keep them informed.

Sometimes children get the idea that they are in the way during a health crisis. If you keep them apprised of what's going on in the hospital and throughout recovery, as well as inform them of the decisions you and your mate are considering, they will feel more included and freer to ask questions.

Children often repeat the same questions over and over again. This does not mean that you've failed to give an appropriate answer or that your child is not listening. Rather, it can be a thermometer for you to gauge your child's anxiety level. Remember, anxiety can play havoc with mental functions, such as concentration, memory, listening, and integration of information.

> Questions for which you have no definite answers are distressing. It is okay to respond with three simple words, "I don't know." Acknowledge the validity of your child's questions, even if you don't know the answers, and assure them that you will try to get the information they need.

The most feared and unsettling question is, of course, "Is my dad going to die?" The truth, especially early in the crisis stage, is that you don't know for sure. You might be tempted to cloak the issue and respond only with the data and statistics that you've heard at the hospital. But this very natural and important question needs an answer from your heart as well as your mind. Your response might be, "Chances are, since your dad has lived through the first forty-eight hours after a heart attack, he will recover. I hope so, although I don't know for sure, and even the doctors can't be certain at this time. I know that you're really scared, and I am, too." Such an answer may be followed by a long hug, shared tears, a special prayer. Trust that your children will handle this truth far better than being deceived or put off.

> If you're ready and willing to answer your children's questions, but they're reluctant to ask, remain open and accessible. They may open up in their own time and appreciate that you haven't shut down.

You might tell them more about your response to the situation; you can model a healthy expression of emotions by saying how you feel. You can remind them that you are available if they want to talk or ask questions. But you can't force children to talk about their feelings and concerns. Pressure will only make them more resistant and uncommunicative.

Every child deals with a family crisis in an individual way. You know from your own observation that each of your children is a unique person, with his or her own personal style of coping with difficulty and relating to the family. Some children, for example, are talkative and inquisitive, while others are less verbal but more prone to observation. There is no right or wrong way to be; although, as a parent, you may be more comfortable with some styles than others. Do your best to acknowledge your children's differences without judgment. It also is important to respond supportively to their differing styles of coping with heart disease and the changes it brings to them and to your family.

Our family had a week to plan before my husband's open-heart surgery. Our daughter, Debbie, decided immediately that she wanted to be with me in the hospital. She said she would be unable to concentrate and would find it intolerable to be sitting in school while her dad was being operated on.

Our fifteen-year-old son, Sid, reacted in a very different way. He thought it would be unbearable to sit for hours at the hospital. His preference was to be at school, to be distracted from the surgery.

He worked out an elaborate plan for being informed. His idea was to race home from school and hear the phone ringing as he unlocked the front door. We agreed on the exact minute that I would call, and we synchronized our watches. And that was how he received the news that his dad had come through the surgery successfully.

I was surprised at how differently our two children reacted. I particularly appreciated that each of them knew exactly what they needed on that stressful day.

Your children may tell their close friends about what's happened to them and their family. You know from your own experience that telling and retelling your story is a necessary review that helps you understand and integrate what has happened and what is happening. Your children have a similar need, though their versions of the experience may be very different than yours.

> Don't "correct" your children's reporting of events. Respect their experience. Like you, how they see will change as they mourn, as they retell their stories, and as time passes.

When your children do share their feelings, you may think it's up to you to make them feel better. You don't have the power to do that. Your right responsibility is to be as available and supportive as you can, trusting in your children's capacity to grieve and in their story-telling process. With your love and support, your children will discover their own sense of order, peace, and understanding from this confusing and chaotic experience.

A Special Word to Cardiackids

As a cardiackid, your concerns are different from those of your parents. Perhaps you've been fortunate to have someone outside the family to talk with about the changes that are taking place. Or maybe you feel confused and alone. In either case, I offer you the following information.

You Have a Right to Information

You have a right to know what is happening. You are entitled, no matter how old or young you are, to know your parent's condition and prognosis. The cardiac crisis is just as real for you as anyone else. Your life is affected by your parent's heart disease. *Ask the questions you need answers to.* You may have to ask your parents because you don't have direct access to doctors and other professionals. If you can't get the answers from your parents, ask others in your family: older brothers and sisters, cousins, aunts and uncles.

There are other sources where you can get information, too. The Web may be one of the best resources available to you. Jeeves for Kids <www.jeevesforkids.com>, for example, is a great search engine where you can find simply worded explanations of technical terms and complex issues. For a broader perspective, seek information using the Google search engine <www.google.com>. You may also find other cardiackids if you search for supportive chat rooms or electronic bulletin boards. Remember that not all information on the Web is accurate. Visit credible sites and ask adults to verify information you gather.

It is important to have reasonable expectations about how information can help you. Information doesn't give you answers to some of your questions. Some things, like how recovered your parent will be or how fast your parent will recover, just don't have concrete answers. Such specific outcomes can't even be predicted by doctors. It is still a good idea to ask all the questions you have. Keeping them hidden inside can make you feel lonely and scared. It is very difficult to have to face the reality that you can't know what is going to happen. Time may bring an answer that you couldn't have known days or weeks ago. The changes that time brings may suggest new and different questions. It helps to share your questions aloud and feel the support of others in your family who are also wanting to know.

Accept and Release Your Feelings

Accept your feelings and find healthy and appropriate ways to release them. *All the feelings that you experience are normal.* Most cardiackids have different feelings at different times. You may go back and forth between feeling sad and happy, afraid and anxious, embarrassed and ashamed, helpless and jealous, depressed and ambivalent, angry and guilty. All of these feelings are okay.

If your family is uncomfortable talking about feelings, find other ways to express yourself. Keep a diary or a journal and regularly write about how you feel. Talk with your friends. Search for an adult who will listen to you. Perhaps your favorite teacher, coach, or activity leader will take the time to hear you out. In a situation like this, your special relationship with a grandparent or favorite relative can be good for both of you.

It really is important for you to express your feelings. Keeping them locked inside can freeze the development of your relationships with your family and other people, too.

Resist Blaming and Shaming Yourself

Don't blame or shame yourself for your mother's or father's heart disease. Cardiackids sometimes believe that their behavior caused their parent's illness. *That is not true!* If you blame yourself, you will act overly careful and withhold your feelings, and that won't help anyone. If somebody tells you that you can cause a fatal heart attack by making a lot of noise, or that angering the patient will cause harm, don't believe it. Your feelings and behavior cannot cause another person's heart attack.

The cardiac experience often triggers feelings of shame. If you believe that your parent is damaged or different because of heart disease, you may feel embarrassed by or ashamed of that parent, your family, even of yourself. It's confusing because you also love your parent and feel guilty about having such negative thoughts.

Ambivalent feelings are normal . . . and confusing. But having a disease, or any physical limitation, doesn't make a person less human. All human beings are sacred and deserve love and respect, regardless of their physical appearance or illness. We are all susceptible to illness and shame. (These truths are illustrated in the films *The Elephant Man* [1980], *The Doctor* [1991], *Mask* [1994], and others. Each of these films is worth viewing.)

It Takes Time to Feel Normal Again

It takes a while to return to normal thinking and functioning after a crisis. What's happened may affect you in ways you might not expect. The energy and enthusiasm for life that you've always taken for granted may have disappeared. You may, for example, find it difficult to perform school or other activities long after your parent returns home from the hospital.

It's okay and important to take care of yourself during this time of change and adjustment. Taking good care of yourself may require you to ease some stresses, to lighten your load temporarily. (Resist any temptation that you might have, however, to use the crisis to procrastinate or to get special privileges.)

Plan for more time than usual to do your homework. You may even ask your teachers to temporarily extend your deadlines. If you find that you can't think clearly, don't push yourself. Stop studying for a while and go for a bike ride, shoot some hoops, call a friend, or take a warm shower. When you go back to the books, be gentle with yourself.

Explain what you and your family are going through to coaches or leaders of your other extracurricular activities. Be sure to let spiritual leaders know, too. It's important to tell those who care about you what has happened and how you are adjusting to the changes in your family.

Roles and Responsibilities Will Change

Roles and responsibilities in the family are changed by the cardiac crisis. You may notice that your parents' roles have switched. Your dad, for example, may have taken over the kitchen since your mother's surgery. Your mom may have become more of a disciplinarian since your dad was hospitalized. You probably have witnessed how your parents are struggling with their new and different responsibilities.

As with your parents, you may be aware of the typical roles and responsibilities that you and your brothers and sisters have. If you've had the reputation as the "helpful child" in the family, you may find yourself feeling really wiped out from taking on extra tasks and jobs to help your parents. If you are the "quiet one" in the family, you may find it hard to get the information you need and even harder to talk about how you feel. Most people fall back on their typical roles to get through a crisis. But the cardiac crisis and recovery will probably require you to take on new roles and responsibilities, too.

This may not be the easiest time to experiment with a new way of interacting with your family, but go for it if you can. A crisis is a time when everything is unfamiliar, so it is possible to try new modes of relating. The need to take on new responsibilities may result in you redefining your strengths and even who you are, as an individual and a member of your family. You may have to get up early to shovel before school, for example, or take over the strenuous house maintenance tasks your parent used to do.

New responsibilities, even temporary ones, can make you feel terrific. It is natural to care when your family is in crisis, and you can show some of that by being responsible and helpful. Putting a younger brother to bed, cleaning up the kitchen, or mowing the lawn may be exactly what you want to do to show your caring to your parents. Such tasks are practical and measurable and can show that you can be counted on when so much seems strange and confusing. On the other hand, you may resent having to take on extra responsibility, especially if you don't have any say in the matter or no one acknowledges your efforts.

In a perfect world, all of these changes would be discussed and accepted before they were required. But the world of the cardiac crisis is far from ideal. It is more likely that you are assigned, sometimes without words, responsibilities that may burden you. Do your best to be tolerant of your parents. Realize that you are not alone in feeling that everything is new, awkward, and strange. Everyone in the family is doing their best to learn how to manage this unexpected new reality that includes heart disease.

Use Your Spiritual Resources

Your spiritual faith can be a solid foundation when a crisis makes you feel lost. There are many ways to be connected with God or your higher power. The most common is prayer, but prayer is as individual as the person who is doing the praying. Some people find formal prayer, led by a spiritual leader in a house of worship, the most comforting. Others find that spending time out in nature is a better fit. Appreciating the beauty of earth, water, flowers, woods, or sky, for example, may be the solace your soul needs to heal.

You may already do things that are spiritually nurturing without realizing that they connect you to your sense of spirit. Take advantage of these resources. Spend time outside doing things you love. Express your pent-up feelings into the open air: run through the woods, sit near running water, feel yourself a part of nature. Play music that soothes your soul. Shout your feelings in the shower. Spend quiet time alone or laugh and cry with your friends. Tell your story over and over until it makes sense to you. Find the place inside you that knows you're okay and that you'll continue to be okay whatever happens.

Your goal is not to get this over with; that's impossible. A more realistic goal is to find your moorings again: to be reconnected to yourself, your family, your friends, your community, your spirituality.

Strive to Understand Your Parents

Your parents' differences and different reactions to the crisis increase their tension and can increase the conflict between them. Whether they tell you so or not, you need to know that they, like you, have a range of responses to what's happened. They may feel helpless, out of control, frightened, sad, and angry. They're also trying to understand and adapt to this new reality.

While your parents are trying to heal, they are having many strong feelings. They struggle with their feelings of failure, too. Fathers especially feel they've failed as the family leader when they fall ill. Mothers are disappointed in themselves when they fail to be there for their children.

Sometimes the family feels that, too. It's easy for family members, especially children, to blame their parents. You may be disappointed in and enraged at the parent who betrayed your trust or withdrew the attention and protection that you've always counted on.

If your parents are separated or divorced, you may feel caught in a loyalty bind. You may live with your mother and depend on her to take you to see your father. It's an awkward situation, but one in which you owe it to yourself to do what your heart tells you. Staying close to your cardiac parent is your right, even if you no longer live together. Discuss the situation with both your parents, letting them know that you love them both.

Communicating your feelings about these issues is important. When possible, discuss your feelings with your parents. When it's not, talk to a trusted friend or mentor. Just talking may help you understand better what your parents are experiencing, and your burden may be lifted, too.

You Are Not Responsible for Your Parents
It is not your responsibility to take care of your parents. That's their job. Even though you may want to fix the heart disease and the emotional pain your parents are feeling and reduce the tension that you feel within your family, *you can only change yourself. You can't change other people.*

The deeper questions you must wrestle with concern your own losses and how to heal your pain. You have seen that your parent is mortal, and now, the one thing you thought was secure, isn't. If your parent can die, then nothing in life is for sure. Remember when you realized there was no Santa or Tooth Fairy? Your disappointment and sadness were real then, and they are now, too. You need time and space to mourn the loss of what you believed. Once you do that, you'll be able to build new trust based on what you've experienced. That may lead you to appreciate just how precious your life and your family are.

Remember, healing takes effort and time. Cardiackids need to express their feelings in their own way, and in their own time.

Our son, Sid, a senior in high school, was assigned to write about an event that had influenced his life. Sid rarely communicated his feelings verbally with the family. I had no idea that his father's heart disease had caused so profound a change in him. His essay was proof to me that images and memories need to be expressed if we are to overcome their hold on us. I was awed and moved as I witnessed Sid's love for his dad when Sid read his essay to us.

He Ain't Hercules, He's My Father
by Sid Levin

A soft, placid sheet of snowflakes filled the skies on the cold winter evening. The scream of the ambulance snapped the peaceful hush of the night, but quickly became muffled. The screams remained in my mind long after. The ambulance held my father in its hollows while he fought for his life with a heart attack. Only minutes before, we were all sitting together watching "Monday Night Football." Now my mother, sister, and I were watching the ambulance disappear into the night. Although I had always loved him, I never realized how valuable my father was to me until I almost lost him.

At age fourteen, I "loved" my father because he was my dad; it was no more than the normal feeling a son has for his father. He was my hero, and I looked up to him as a boy does to his favorite sports star. In high school, my father captained three sports: football, basketball, and baseball. He was the "all-city" quarterback and was voted the best athlete by his class. Through his mid-forties he remained physically active, participating in softball, racquetball, and golf. He not only instructed me in the fine points of baseball, he also taught me how to wrestle by pinning me weekly during our "roughhousing matches." From my perspective, he was as close to Hercules as a man could get. I never had a foreshadowing of the disastrous event.

The hospital room was only steps away. I slowed my pace, afraid to see my wounded father. I peeked in and saw him: lifeless, with tubes going into and out of his body. His eyes opened when I entered the room, and when he made an effort to smile, I broke into tears. I could not believe that my hero was crippled. He was too weak to lift his hand to hold mine, so I grasped his hand and I held him, all of him, for the first time in my life. At that point, I realized how much I loved him! He was a supernova, an exploded star that had become thousands of times stronger and brighter.

After his hospitalization, my father returned home and didn't leave the house for another month. His body had failed him; as time passed, he started to adjust. I learned what true disappointment was by watching the pain that he went through; it hurt inside to see him short of breath after climbing a flight of stairs.

With my hero gone, a new relationship with my father dawned. Because of the threat that any day he could be gone forever, I have learned to value his presence whenever I am with him. I no longer take his "being there" for granted. No more do I worship my father as a hero. Rather, I observe with new eyes and have a greater understanding of who he really is. I watch him make mistakes, and I note his shortcomings. We discuss our daily lives, share humor, and compare our beliefs. My hero is gone. But I have a deeper feeling of love for the man that took his place.

Helping Your Children Heal

Honoring the fact that every cardiackid has his or her own experience is a way to help them heal. As parents we can only marvel at our children's courage and resilience, watching their pain transform to love as they learn about mortality and the preciousness of family and of life.

Although your children are different from you, and each of them is unique, all of you will go through a similar process.

> Universally, family members experience disruption, shock, confusion, anxiety, fear, depression, and anger, and eventually adapt to a new family life that includes heart disease.

Everyone may exhibit and express their reactions differently, but each of you is grieving and recovering from this family crisis.

Children need to be encouraged to speak about the frightening images they have. Like telling a nightmare, bringing the dark and terrifying memories into the light may divest them of their power, even if they are never forgotten.

When given the opportunity, most cardiackids are eager to talk about their experiences and images. One young man said that he couldn't get free from the horrible image of his mom straining against the respirator. A teenager described her pain and shock at seeing her father so vulnerable in the cardiac care unit after a heart attack.

An adult cardiackid explained his paralysis in the family business. He imagined his father, the perfect businessman, connected everywhere to life-giving tubes, weakly shaking his head no at every business decision the son considered. He was sure that he would make an irreversible mistake. He had to confront his feelings of inadequacy as he moved toward the inevitable: the younger generation taking over the work of the patriarch.[2]

Cardiac families rarely talk about how the patient looked after open-heart surgery. The sounds of the respirator and the numerous monitoring devices; the sight of countless tubes coming in and going out of the patient's body, neck, and nose; the antiseptic smells and the chill of the patient's flesh are too much to assimilate. The technology may be sophisticated, and the techniques may be routine, but when adults or children of any age see a loved one in this state, they often respond with horror, terror, or despair. If the unspoken rule is to say nothing or "keep a stiff upper lip," each family member suffers silently with disturbing memories and images.

A mother expressed concern that for months her nine-year-old son, Bobby, cried every time he heard an ambulance siren. It was suggested she ask Bobby what the sound reminded him of, and that she respond to him from her heart. Bobby told her that the sound reminded him of seeing his daddy being taken away in the dark night by a screaming ambulance. He didn't think he would ever see his dad again. Bobby sat on his mom's lap and they had a long hug. Then they talked about how scary that time had been for everyone in the family, and how lucky they all were that Dad had recovered. Happily, after their talk, the gripping power of Bobby's memory began to fade.

Sharing your feelings with your children can be a relief for all of you. There is no need to hide your honest emotions. Expressing your feelings openly is an act of courage, one that may give your children permission to do the same. Shared family tears soothe and heal.

Children in cardiac families, especially younger children, may need an expanded foundation of support during the cardiac crisis.

> If you have school-age children, tell their teachers and other significant adults about the cardiac crisis. The information will help adults recognize your children's experience, understand changes in behavior, and identify their special needs.

Teachers can symbolize stability during times of confusion and change. An adult ally outside the family can be a child's best source of support.

Carla visited her daughters' parochial school when Matthew needed open-heart surgery. She wanted the teachers to be prepared for their girls' reactions. Carla was pleasantly surprised to find that her eight-year-old, Marie, had already told her teacher. In fact, she had asked that a special prayer for her dad be included in the daily morning prayer. Next, Carla visited her ten-year-old's teacher. The teacher knew nothing about the family crisis and was glad to be aware so she could be helpful. Carla returned home confident that the girls' teachers, now informed, would do what they could to listen and provide reassurance without minimizing the girls' concerns.

Informing teachers may include educating them about heart disease and telling them that this is a family crisis, even though recovery is expected. Open-heart surgery has come to be seen as routine; with over 500 bypass operations done every day in the United States, it is our most common surgery. As the frequency of angioplasty procedures surpasses surgery, we grow even more accustomed to thinking of these treatments as ordinary. Recovering from a heart attack is often thought only to be an occasion for celebration and gratitude. Talking with teachers will help them understand the seriousness of the situation.

It is important to note that despite the love and support they receive, children, like adults, sometimes get stuck in their grief and recovery. Because each child is unique, it is not easy to define normal progress. You know your child better than anyone. If you sense that he or she is having serious problems, trust your judgment and seek help.

The following are generally accepted as universal warning signals for unresolved grief or problems coping with major change. Some of these behaviors, if short in duration, are normal for children who are grieving or in crisis. (Note that alcohol or drug problems are never normal.) When determining whether to seek assistance, take into account how long a particular behavior continues and how your child's behaviors have changed since the cardiac crisis began.

- Alcohol or drug problems
- Angry or rebellious outbursts
- Asking the same questions over and over
- Bedwetting
- Behavior problems at school
- Belligerent or argumentative behavior
- Clinging to parents
- Crippling fears
- Dramatic drop in school grades
- Eating or sleeping problems

- Lethargy or exhaustion
- Persistent nightmares
- Uncontrollable crying
- Withdrawal or isolation

If you believe your child is suffering from any of these behaviors, consult the school social worker, a crisis or grief counselor, or a psychologist. Another resource is your local hospital's social service department. You may find professionally led programs available to your child at school or at the hospital. Many high schools have groups for students who are experiencing unexpressed grief or family stress. Expert advice doesn't supplant your influence; it supplements it.

Here is a guide to help you evaluate your family members' needs as they deal with the crisis. It includes reminders and hints to improve communication within the family. You will also find suggestions for getting help and support for your family.

HEARTMATES®
FAMILY NEEDS ASSESSMENT GUIDE

1. Does each family member know that it is normal for the entire family to be affected when one member has heart disease? If not, how can such an understanding come about?
- Get more information.
- Ask more questions.
- Have more discussion among family members.
- Express feelings.
- Share this guide, chapter, or book with family members.

2. How aware and supportive are you of each child's reaction to the cardiac crisis? (Think about the initial and long-range reactions of each family member.) Here is the perfect moment to value and appreciate the uniqueness of each member of your family.

3. Do family members ask questions and express concerns that are important to them individually? Here are some suggestions to help relax the code of silence if it exists in your family:

- At your next family dinner or meeting, ask directly if anyone has questions about your spouse's present condition, past cardiac events, or future plans.
- Establish a question box in the kitchen that can be opened regularly at a time when all family members are present. Let questions be asked in writing, anonymously, for family members who are reticent to voice their concerns.
- Be willing to share your questions, too. You don't have to understand everything perfectly. Other family members may be able to offer new perspectives, and they'll appreciate that you're human, too.

4. How do you inform your children about the difficulties you are having?

- Do you say how you feel?
- Do you ask them to listen to you?
- Do you solicit their opinions and advice as you confront necessary and difficult decisions?
- Do you allow your children to give to you physically, emotionally, financially?

5. Does each family member have someone outside the family to talk to regarding the cardiac crisis? Is the listener available often, regularly, or seldom? Is the listener an extended family member, a friend of approximately the same age, a special adult, a mentor, a spiritual guide?

6. Have you asked others outside the family for support?

- Encourage family members to help make a list of family needs and potential resources. Decide who can best make each contact, and delegate the work.
- Inform your children's teachers.
- Let your spiritual or religious leader know of your family crisis.
- Contact your hospital cardiac rehabilitation social service staff.
- Seek help from a social service agency or a family therapist specializing in family concerns, grief, or crises.

Simply wanting your family to become more intimate isn't enough to make it happen. Family patterns are established over long periods of time, often passed down through generations. Consequently, change is slow, one step at a time. Even positive change includes an element of uncertainty, so it can be strange and, in some ways, rather frightening.

During the process of recovery, anything uncertain can feel threatening. Go slowly. Remember that you alone are not responsible for all the other members of your family. As much as you may hope that this crisis will be a catalyst for closeness, you can't make other people change and you can't fix them. Concentrate on how *you* can be rightly responsible, available to give and receive from members of your family.

The Nontraditional Family

Heart disease does not confine itself to traditional families. It strikes separated and divorced couples, blended families, and unmarried partners. Adapting to these complex situations becomes even more challenging when heart disease and recovery are added to the mix. Lack of clarity about whether you are part of a family when you are separated, divorced, or in a second marriage is a serious question lacking formal guidelines. The answer varies from family to family. In the wake of love and clashing loyalties, children experience confusion and uncertainty. They question the legitimacy of their feelings and don't know what they should do. Events that have an impact on families, and surely heart disease is one of these, mark all family members, former and current.

Families of Separation and Divorce

As a former spouse of a heart patient, your concerns will run the gamut from responding emotionally to his heart disease to wondering how to help your children. You probably have at least some of the following questions: Should I visit at the hospital? Why do I feel sad, angry, or afraid when we're no longer married? Is it appropriate for me to share my feelings with the patient? With our children? How should I act in relation to his family? How can I interact with his present spouse? What is the most supportive position I can take for our children in a family crisis from which I'm isolated, or about which I have unresolved feelings?

Act from your heart and use your best judgment. There are no right or wrong answers.

> There is no etiquette book or protocol that can help you discover what's best for you and your family. Each situation is unique. If there is anything unresolved between you and your former spouse, there may be criticism no matter what you do.

Try not to judge or censor your feelings. Ambivalence is normal in this situation. You may find that the crisis and recovery offer the opportunity to examine feelings and reconcile old differences. This is perfectly appropriate. Hurts may ease and resentments soften when heart disease has made all of you more vulnerable. It's important to understand, however, that nothing may change between you and your former spouse or that the situation and your feelings may be further complicated by the illness.

But no matter how you feel toward your former spouse, do your best to respect your children's relationships with him. If your children's loyalty has been a point of contention, a family health crisis can escalate it. Your children's love should not be fought over or used as a tool to express resentments. Children should never have to shoulder the extra burden of your unresolved issues. *They have a right to their own personal relationship with each of you.*

If you feel unwelcome or too awkward to visit the patient at the hospital or at home during recovery, call a member of your former spouse's family to pass along your best sentiments and to arrange visits for your young children. Encourage older children to follow their hearts in making decisions about visiting. Be truthful about the health of the patient and the situation so they can make informed decisions.

When you have unresolved feelings about your former spouse or your separation, you may find that you can't help your children with aspects of the crisis and recovery. You can't "be there" for them.

> It is hard to accept that your children need some-
> thing that you aren't in a position to give. But being
> a good parent doesn't mean you can meet their
> every need.

You can be there for them in other ways. You might, for example, arrange for them to connect with grandparents or aunts and uncles who can function as confidants, providing the steady support and affection required in such a difficult situation.

Blended Families

Support is especially needed when there are unresolved issues in blended families coping with heart disease.

> Blended families have all the complex dynamics of
> divorced and separated families, with the addi-
> tional complication of stepparents and sometimes
> stepsiblings.

If you have children or teens, yours or his, living under the same roof, the conditions and difficulties are different than if the children are grown and no longer living with you.

You may be disappointed to see that your children are less affected by the illness than his are. You may find it hard to understand, especially when you have worked hard to unify the family. In order to be fair to the children, you need to be realistic. You have not failed. You love your mate and your children. The fact that your children may be struggling with conflicting loyalties between their father and their stepfather is not something you can or should try to control.

You may also question whether you can be as comforting to your husband's children as their mother. It helps if you have a cooperative relationship with your mate's former spouse. Together you can create a loving, supportive environment to enable the children to heal.

When your former mate is the person who has heart disease, your children may wonder if it is okay with you that they love their father. It can be confusing for everyone. A rule of thumb is to honor all feelings as legitimate. Remember, each family member will have his or her own feelings about the situation, and the family will heal best when everyone receives respect for how they feel. When they do, they will have permission to act in accordance with their feelings and their best judgment.

For the grown children of blended families, the complications continue. Adult children are affected by the heart disease of their parent, too. Though they may have been independent, perhaps building their own families for years, they are still cardiackids. But who are their parents? How many parents do they have? What are their responsibilities in relationship with the current spouse of their parent, who they may not know well or have an intimate relationship with? How might this complicate their relationship with their well parent? Do cardiackids expect to be treated differently by their parent's current spouse because their parent is ill? Does their parent expect support from them when the current spouse becomes ill? The questions go on and on. They suggest common concerns for which there are *no right answers*.

From the "Interactive Connections Archive" page on the Heartmates Web site, here is a heartfelt expression of grief and confusion, a call for support, from a woman in a second marriage:

> *I need a little support right now, even though nothing is seriously wrong at the moment. My husband has cardiomyopathy. He is doing fairly well at the moment, but since I have a medical background in this area, I know his prognosis.*
>
> *I know that I will be facing life alone in the not-too-distant future and wish I could talk over my options with my best friend. But, as my husband is my best friend, I can't do that because I don't want to upset him.*
>
> *My children live in another state, as do his; this is our second marriage and we have no children together, so it is not easy to talk to them about it. Any suggestions?*

All heartmates, including those in divorced, separated, and blended families, want and need support and healing for themselves and their loved ones. Although each situation and every family is unique, there are some things that work universally. First, respect your feelings and the unique feelings of all family members, then express them.

> Communicating your feelings, needs, and stories is one side of the coin; the other is to have someone who will listen to you.

Often, answers about what to do will come from within after you talk about what is happening.

Writing in your journal is important, too, potentially opening you to your deepest self. Praying to the God of your understanding may also help your family to heal. If your issues feel too overwhelming to address alone, within your family, or within your circle of support, seek the counsel of a professional therapist or your spiritual mentor.

Unmarried Heartmates

If you are an unmarried heartmate, your situation poses questions of a different sort. Heartmate relationships take a variety of shapes, including companions, people planning to marry in the future, people who have chosen not to marry, and couples for whom marriage is not possible. Whatever your situation, there are questions about how you, as a heartmate, are accepted by the family of the heart patient. If you are not considered to be part of the family, you may face additional difficulties in supporting each other through the cardiac crisis and recovery. Some heartmates find their grief and healing complicated by legal and financial concerns beyond their control.

Family members who rally round your sick mate may not think of you as part of the family. They may fail to recognize the importance of including you when discussing plans and decisions about the patient. In some cases, the family may not realize the significance of your relationship or even know that your relationship exists. They may neither appreciate the nature of your relationship nor realize that you are deeply affected by your mate's illness.

If your relationship has been a secret from the family, your contact may need to be clandestine or temporarily cut off. This secret, previously painful, now may feel unbearable. Since heart disease is incurable—and potentially life-threatening, even when recovery is complete—this crisis may be a catalyst for a change in your relationship. You may decide that it's worth going public and risking your families' nonacceptance or disapproval.

Once the secret's out, you may be surprised by your families' reactions. The crisis of heart disease may open channels of compassion and understanding. A family's values may shift, allowing for acceptance, inclusion, and honest intimacy. Love may flow freely.

In some cases, however, all the discussion in the world, all the yearning for acceptance, will not make it happen. You may need to come to terms with grieving and adapting without the safety and support of your families.

Financial arrangements for your future also may need to be revisited. A health crisis can give rise to new values, affecting the way you deal with money in your relationship. Your financial situation may change if your partner is forced to cut back on work, whether temporarily or permanently.

> Whatever your situation, you suffer during the cardiac crisis, as all heartmates do. Your feelings and your caring for each other need to be respected.

Seek people who can support you, who will listen compassionately to your experience and concerns. Professional counseling may be a practical aid when your needs require confidentiality.

Getting Your Family Unstuck, Not Unglued

When a family gets stuck in the process of recovery, when communication is essentially shut off so that issues are not being confronted, when secrets are choking the family, then the emotional, psychological, and even physical healing process is delayed or prevented. Grief and mourning go unresolved.

A "stuck" family may look like this one: Several months of recovery have passed. Father, the cardiac patient, is depressed, irritable, and demanding. Mother, the cardiac spouse, is resentful, overworked, and fatigued. The eldest daughter, who temporarily dropped out of college when her father suffered his heart attack, has neither looked for a job nor made arrangements to continue her schooling. The second child, a sixteen-year-old high school junior, is coming home late at night. His sullen and silent style has become exaggerated, and his grades have plummeted. The youngest child, an eleven-year-old girl, is afraid to go to bed without a light on, and is often heard crying or screaming with nightmares. No one comments on what is happening to anyone in the family. No one mentions that the family as a unit is failing its members. The crisis seems to have fragmented the family system, with adults and children acting out their neglected pain and grief indirectly. They start to blame one another, relegating symptoms of family dysfunction to individual family members. The son with falling grades, for example, is misperceived as lazy, unfocused, or a troublemaker. His real needs go unmet, which leaves him feeling abandoned and misunderstood. No member of the family feels safe, nurtured, supported, or loved.

This example underscores the dangers of denial, secrecy, and suppression. It is indicative of a family that needs help facing and coping with its issues. Members of the family in this example are shut down and cut off from one another. A family therapist, in short-term consultation, can encourage the cardiac couple to take the lead in directly facing and dealing with their issues. This establishes a new system of openness, support, and nurturance, liberating the parents and their children. Brief intervention is frequently all a "stuck" family needs to break through their code of silence.

Through the leadership and example of the cardiac couple, the parents, any family can work to prevent getting stuck.

> When parents are able to relate their feelings
> about heart disease and the cardiac experience in
> healthy ways, it has magical effects for all family
> members.

Family members see that it is okay to open up and share their pain. When they acknowledge their difficult feelings as well as their positive ones, the chance that their hearts will open to each other increases exponentially, and the family can become a secure and healing place for everyone. Healing—recovery—is built on a foundation of safety, trust, respect, and love.

Visualization is one technique you can use to promote the safe and healthy expression of feelings and issues. The following is a guided visualization exercise that you can do on your own, then share with your family. Another option is to do the exercise together. If you first do the exercise by yourself, tape the instructions and play them back to guide your visualization. As a family, you can either tape the instructions or take turns being the guide. Whether you speak the instructions directly or tape them, make sure you pause as indicated to allow each family member time to reflect.

HEARTMATES®
VISUALIZATION: A FAMILY MEETING

Find a quiet and comfortable place to sit. When you are settled, read or play back these instructions:

Close your eyes. Let yourself breathe normally. . . . Imagine that with each inhalation you breathe in healing energy and peace, and with each exhalation you let go of tension. . . . Let go of any distractions cluttering your mind. . . . Continue to focus on your breathing until you feel relaxed and alert. . . .

Now imagine a room in your home that is the coziest and most comfortable for you or your family. It may be your kitchen, den, or porch. . . . See it awaiting and welcoming your family. Notice its furnishings, those things that make it warm and inviting. . . . In your mind's eye, see all your family seated in a circle in this comfortable room. . . . Everyone seems to know why they're here. The atmosphere is hopeful and cooperative.

You begin your family meeting with everyone holding hands. Together you share a silent prayer of gratitude for recovery and a petition for family cohesion and individual strength. . . . As much as you can, allow yourself to experience how it feels with all of you together in this moment of silence. . . . As you complete the prayer, everyone drops hands, and an atmosphere of respect and concern settles over the room. A peace, a sense of acceptance and protection, blankets the family. . . .

Now imagine that each family member, without blame or shame, speaks in turn about one personal concern. . . . You listen with your heart to what each family member says. . . . You, in turn, hear your own contribution with your heart as well. . . . There is no verbal response to any statement that is made, but there is respect in the listening, and there is caring from each to all.

Imagine that as each person speaks, the weight of the family is lightened and the light in the room gets brighter. . . . The air the family is breathing is fresh and clean. . . . You can smell scents pleasing to you, fresh-mown grass, blossoming flowers. . . .

Now, as the meeting ends, you sense family members really seeing one another. . . . Members are respectful of each other's right and ability to deal with the crisis in their own way and on their own timetable. . . . Some affection may be expressed. . . . Everyone agrees to meet again soon. As you leave this favorite room, you each experience realistic hope about your family's ability to cope with and heal from the cardiac crisis. . . .

You again focus your attention on your own breath. . . . Gradually return to your present reality. . . . Continue to breathe fully and naturally. . . . Stand up and be aware of the floor supporting you. . . . Gently and slowly return, renewed, to the present.

The purpose of doing the guided meditation or consulting with a family therapist is to further healing. What works for one family may not work for another. Keep in mind that the goal is to renew respect and hope among family members. Once members feel heard and understood, their resilience shows up. Family members can pull together in difficult times, and the family can build on an environment of inclusion within which members can grieve, heal, and get their needs met.

Recovery and Hope for the Cardiac Family

How can you see opportunity in the cardiac crisis? "In the light of our everyday world, we cannot see the stars."[3] So much of your energy goes into coping with the minute-to-minute and day-to-day changes, to longing for the way things were or for a normal future, to surviving, adjusting, and accepting—to grieving. The stars of healing may be difficult to see at first, but, as you heal, you will come to see their light.

The power of the crisis jolted and shocked each of you and wounded the family. Everyone needs to recover, individually and as a family unit. What can you do? Recovery and healing are a natural part of a crisis. The essential elements of every recovery include time, telling "your" story, communicating, expressing feelings, and nurturing one another through the grieving process. Together you can move toward understanding and accepting the changes in your lives.

> Make space for everyone's recovery to unfold within the loving and protective embrace of the family.

The crisis has different consequences for each family member. The pace of a family's healing is also unique. Your family will move at its own rate and in its own way toward recovery. Build an environment with and for one another that honors individual differences and permits each person his or her own responses. Being there for one another puts "heart" into the family.

Chapter 9 Notes

1. See Dr. David Keith's case study in the foreword of this book.

2. See "How Devastating Illness Devastates the Family," in Maggie Strong's *Mainstay: For the Well Spouse of the Chronically Ill* (Boston: Little, Brown, & Co., 1988).

3. Jean Shinoda Bolen, MD, *The Tao of Psychology, Synchronicity, and the Self* (San Francisco: Harper & Row, 1979), 2.

10

Opening Your Heart: Finding Meaning and Connection

The experience of the cardiac crisis may seem to you mainly a matter of coping. Six months, a year, even five years down the road you may remember this as a time when you took care of business and bumbled along the best you knew how. The countless adjustments, from medical decisions to lifestyle changes, consumed your energy, attention, and time.

Feeling needy and self-centered—cocooning—is a normal, instinctive act of self-protection during the acute period of crisis and the early stages of recovery. Your world got very tiny while you were preoccupied with your personal issues.

In 1977, a friend recommended that I read the book, Alive, *a true story about the survivors of a plane crash in South America. I didn't recall ever hearing or reading about the crash in the news. Opening the book, I was surprised to find that the date of the crash was the same day as my mother's funeral. At first I felt embarrassed about being so out of step, and I wondered what else I'd missed, being so absorbed in my personal pain. But when I thought about it, I understood the natural tendency for energy to flow where it is most needed. I imagine it's the same when white cells rush to a wound at a specific location in the body to provide the additional help needed for healing.*

As you heal, you have a real opportunity to emerge from your cocoon, "reconnect," and expand your world. Recovery might be defined as the gradual process of moving back into relationship with the larger world around you. This is similar to the developmental stages children go through as their world expands to include loyalty to and trust in their family, their friends, then their school, community, state, country, and, hopefully, planet.

As you emerge, like a chrysalis awaiting transformation to a butterfly, you may experience dissatisfaction, restlessness, and an urge to find new meaning in your life. Questions about the deeper life changes signal the final stop on the road to recovery. They're different from the questions you've dealt with regarding changes in diet, exercise, lifestyle, or family concerns. Modern-day ethicist Daniel C. Maguire suggests that just as the body needs oxygen, the mind and soul need meaning.[1] These questions, spiritual in nature, born out of an unexpected and disruptive crisis, are the guideposts pointing to a new perspective, a new foundation of meaning.

The Healing Heart

Before Reid's open-heart surgery, everything in Susan's life was perfect. A forty-year-old interior decorator, mother of two, and self-described optimist, Susan always maintained a positive attitude, no matter what problems she confronted. In the first few weeks following Reid's heart surgery, she carried on with her usual buoyancy and enthusiasm. "He's doing great, couldn't be better!" Susan would respond to all queries about Reid's health.

One afternoon, while Reid napped, Susan turned on the television just in time to see a public service announcement about heart disease. Suddenly she was crying. She felt as if her heart were breaking. Tears flowing, Susan began to feel her disappointment, exhaustion, and fear. She was sick to death of pretending that everything was fine. In that split second, she gave herself permission to be vulnerable and human, to grieve.

From that moment forward, Susan's life, including the consequences of Reid's heart disease, contained a new element, the potential for new and richer meaning. Another heartmate clearly expressed
this potential in her own words: "I've been transformed by heart disease . . . if I had to go back to being the person I was before all this
happened, I'd choose it again."

The following is an excerpt from a poem, a holiday message of gratitude for friends and family, written by a cardiac spouse, Kathy. Her
words capture the cardiac experience from beginning to end or, more
accurately, from the end of what was to the new beginning of what is.

Some Lessons Well-Learned from a Heart Attack

. . . A beautiful summer . . . morning . . . turns into a tempest—
A . . . flood of disbelief, shock, surreal numbness, of fear—
. . . an internist and cardiologist who gave Dick the best of their
science and me the whole of their art—
. . . Your children all of a sudden fully graduated from childhood to
adulthood—
. . . Trust, hope, surrender, only words before—
. . . Long, scary days . . .
Prayers . . . and nights . . . beeping monitors . . . long-distance
phone calls—
. . . Time and healing—
. . . Ups and downs, gradually more on the upside—
. . . The fragility of life—
. . . There is still fear—
A certain innocence is gone—
Yet there is joy and appreciation of the present as never before—
And so many more trout streams to explore!
I know now what is meant . . . in the darkest of times you can see
God most clearly—
. . . Join us in our resounding yes to life.[2]

Spirituality and Prayer

Kathy's poem might be considered a prayer. Prayer takes many forms. Traditional liturgical prayers of a faith tradition meet the needs of some people who are ill or in crisis. Other people find meaning and connection in their own spontaneous creative expressions. Some people pray silently within their hearts; others whisper, sing, or even shout from mountaintops. Some people pray aloud whether they are in solitude or in community.

Every part of our world is sacred or can be made sacred by our prayers, whether we pray in hospital waiting rooms, in awesome settings of nature, in sanctuaries, in our cars, or in our homes. Prayers may be intimate conversations with God. They may be petitions, requests for healing, for peace, for safety, for acceptance, for the strength to continue, for the courage to carry out a higher power's will today. Prayers may also be expressions of gratitude for the blessings of life, for being. Prayer is a means by which we ask a power greater than ourselves to assist us in our need for connection and understanding.

Recent studies in healthcare indicate the efficacy of prayer and religious affiliation. All of the major faiths have revived the tradition of healing services, incorporating prayers for the sick and their caregivers. Regular attendance at faith services has been found to reduce cardiovascular deaths by 50 percent, according to Stanford psychologist Fred Luskin, PhD (as reported in his keynote address to cardiac rehabilitation professionals in 1999).[3]

Viktor Frankl, a philosopher and World War II concentration camp survivor, wrote: "Man's main concern is not to gain pleasure or to avoid pain but rather to see a meaning in his life. That is why man is even ready to suffer, on the condition, to be sure, that his suffering has a meaning."[4] Heartmates know they are in the final stage of recovery when their focus naturally shifts to seeking the meaning in what they have experienced. This is the time when you may experience being blessed, having a sense of purpose, and wanting to help others. This is the spiritual dimension of recovery and healing.

Finding Meaning in Adversity

The cardiac crisis and recovery challenge our understanding of our world, our lives, even our faith. Valerie, a fifty-eight-year-old spouse, came to her marriage with a strong religious background. Her spiritual activities gave her pleasure and meaning. She established her family's routine to include church and regular evening prayer. She taught Sunday school and was active in church activities.

After Walter's heart attack, Valerie felt that God had abandoned her. She wrestled with the question, "If there's a God, how could He allow this to happen?" She analyzed her life, trying to understand why she "deserved" such bad treatment. Her faith challenged, she turned away from the God she had trusted since childhood. Valerie resigned from her job as Sunday school teacher and, for a while, stopped attending church with her family.

Valerie's crisis of faith helped her to deepen her spirituality. Questioning ideas that she had accepted blindly as a child eventually led Valerie to a renewed faith and a deeper understanding of God, herself, and her world. She began to understand that Walter's heart attack was not about God punishing her or Walter. She gradually came to accept that difficulties, disease, even suffering are part of the human condition. With that understanding, Valerie's faith matured, and she returned to her relationship with God.

In *At the Will of the Body,* Arthur W. Frank writes about his discoveries as a heart patient, ideas that are applicable to heartmates as well:

> *Illness [crisis] takes away parts of your life, but in doing so it gives you the opportunity to choose the life you will lead, as opposed to living out the one you have simply accumulated over the years.*[5]

Crisis offers us an awakening. We can no longer count on all that we once took for granted.

I wouldn't have wished heart disease on my spouse, or anyone. But it certainly woke me up. Our marriage and our lives had settled into a comfortably predictable pattern. Married for more than twenty years, we had long ago lost the sense of mystery and excitement that earlier had marked our relationship. We knew each other well, had learned to sidestep our differences, and over time had softened the rough edges of our relationship. We had deepened the groove by long habit and had reached a point where we took each other for granted, not the sort of atmosphere in which growth blossoms. We had reached the "flabby forties." We were settled down and settled in.

Coming to terms with the idea of a limited quantity of life opens the heartmate to consider the unlimited quality of life. Your experience results in a series of deep personal questions about your values, priorities, and beliefs. Your relationship with your mate, your family, your higher power or God, and your own soul are suddenly significant and genuine concerns.

We're often blind to changes within us. Beth, a thirty-year-old cardiac spouse, experienced what she described as a surprising need for spiritual support. In the middle of the night before Gary's surgery, she awoke with a start. She was terrified and shaking. She tried telling herself that everything was all right and that he'd make it through the operation. But she couldn't silence her fears.

Beth got out of bed and walked outside where she stood alone in the dark beneath the stars. Suddenly she began to pray. Although Beth had never thought of herself as religious, her prayer was the comfort she needed at that moment. Opening her soul on that dark night was the beginning of faith for Beth, a faith that translated into a new career. She completed a training course for chaplains and now works with cardiac families at a metropolitan hospital.

Beth's story illustrates how personal experience can translate into a more meaningful life, a commitment to work to help make things better, to express one's faith in action. In *Fire in the Soul,* Joan Borysenko writes, "Each wound we suffer and eventually heal from is a soul-making experience with the potential to awaken our willingness to participate in the healing of the world."[6]

Allow your heart to open, and let it guide your life. Following your heart can transform day-to-day activities and relationships into an authentic celebration of life.

Spirituality and Service

Not everyone finds a new career or makes dramatic life changes as a result of a health crisis. A Zen monk explained to the wood gatherer and water carrier that after enlightenment they would still gather wood and carry water. From the ones who gather wood and carry water to the ones who do laundry and make dinner, each of us has a purpose. It's not what we do but how we do it that makes our lives mundane or meaningful.

Serving others because you think you should or you feel obligated to "be good" is draining and exhausting. Authentic service, on the other hand, is a natural human tendency.[7] We are spontaneously drawn to do service. It is the natural outpouring of the human heart that, paradoxically, nourishes the one who is giving as much as those receiving.

Until I was forty, I spent most of my energy trying to "do good" without knowing why. In retrospect, I know I believed I was bad; the only way to hide my shadow from others and earn their love was to be a do-gooder.

I was sure that someone other than I knew the right way to "do good," and I was determined to learn how. I experimented with various forms of yoga, diets, meditations, and therapy. I read every self-help book I could get my hands on. I studied psychology and even shifted careers, leaving teaching to become a therapist. I hoped that by helping others, I might get fixed, too.

I was a continual disappointment to myself. My feet would fall asleep as I tried to sit in the lotus position. I was nauseated, not enlightened, by the odor of incense. I always felt like a fraud or a failure when I applied someone else's answers to my life questions. It was like wearing someone else's shoes that pinched because they were too tight, made me trip because they were too wide, or, worst of all, didn't match my outfit.

One evening, about a year after my mate's open-heart surgery, I accepted an invitation to a meditation service led by a Tibetan lama. I arrived a few minutes late and sat down in the back of a room filled with chanting Americans. At first I was absorbed, not by the holiness or the mystery, but by my curiosity: how many Westerners were stuffed into this room, all shoeless, seated in uncomfortable poses? (If I could even sit in the posture, at my age and with my sedentary lifestyle, my body would be sore the next day for sure.) Some were chanting in a unified response to the lama, who was draped in an orange-red robe and whose head was shaved. I could hear my grandfather: "What's a nice Jewish girl doing in a place like this?"

I myself wondered what I was doing there. I recalled the many evenings I had spent similarly, leaving my family, racing off to hear a speaker, an author, a teacher, a guru. And always I returned home disappointed, never finding the answers I had hoped for.

I started to think about what I had done in the past that had given me satisfaction. I recalled how meaningful it had been to create a hospital program for the families of dying patients in the early 1970s. I knew of the need for the program because of my experience there when my mother died.

My work with heartmates had come from my own heart as well. I felt great empathy for the unrecognized suffering and lack of support for heartmates everywhere.

Sitting in that room, while everyone chanted, I began to understand. What is spiritual for me is participating in the human activity of "making things better." (My faith, Judaism, defines service as tikkun olam, "healing the world.")

I have begun the spiritual journey: to accept myself, to forgive myself for being me, not someone else or someone better. I have begun to feel awe and gratitude for my life and my gifts. I am me, a precious, sacred human, made in the image of God, vulnerable, and, darn it, fallible (even acceptance is imperfect!), enjoying the struggle to find meaning and purpose and God. And that, I believe, is what God wants of me.

This doesn't mean that I forget my previous experience, but it does mean that I don't make myself a bad person for my past. As I have become more forgiving of myself, I have become more empathic and compassionate toward others I used to judge and fear.[8] I've found and will continue to find ways, born from my personal experience, to do my part to heal the world. I already have something to offer, something to give, something that can help. I don't have to don foreign clothes, assume uncomfortable postures, or eat weird foods to feel good about myself or to have a meaningful life. All I have to do is stay open, trust God, and respond to the opportunities presented in my own life.

As I continue to do "my work," I celebrate life by giving something back to the world.⁹ I have been richly blessed, and I have suffered. I no longer yearn to study one more discipline, or feel tempted to hit the circuit for one more lecture.

It's still somewhat unsettling to acknowledge that I am at peace with myself, my life, my spirituality. But each time I do, I know more surely that the way of my own heart is a spiritual way. At the same time, I'm learning to be more tolerant of others whose journeys are very different from mine. They're searching for their unique paths and trying to understand the meaning of their lives.

I hope you will be blessed, as I have been, with increased choices, a realistic hope for the future, and a deeper connection to self, others, and the God of your understanding. Heart disease need not be an end. It can, in fact, usher in a new and fulfilling beginning for your mate, for your family, and for you.

Chapter 10 Notes

1. From a 1993 lecture in Minneapolis by Daniel C. Maguire, professor of ethics at Marquette University and author of *The Moral Core of Judaism and Christianity* (Philadelphia: Fortress Press, 1993).
2. Kathy Hanousek can be contacted through the Heartmates Web site. Write to her on the "Interactive Connection" page at <www.heartmates.com>.
3. Fred Luskin, PhD, director of the Stanford Forgiveness Project, author of *Forgive for Good* (New York: HarperCollins, 2001).
4. Viktor E. Frankl, MD, *The Doctor and the Soul* (New York: Vintage, 1955). See especially the sections "The Meaning of Life" and "The Meaning of Suffering."
5. Arthur W. Frank, *At the Will of the Body* (Boston: Houghton-Mifflin, 1991). A sensitive and beautifully written account of Frank's experience as a heart and cancer patient. His appreciation of his spouse, his anguish when he's unable to protect her from being ignored by the healthcare professionals, is a strong component of the book, one that is particularly healing for heartmates. Frank shows what it's like to survive two life-threatening illnesses before age forty.

6. Joan Borysenko, PhD, *Fire in the Soul: A New Psychology of Spiritual Optimism* (New York: Warner Books, 1993). I recommend this book because of its usefulness to people beginning to seriously explore their spirituality apart from religious institutions.

7. See the Service section in John Firman and James Vargiu's article "Dimensions of Growth," in *Synthesis* vol. 3–4 (Redwood City, Calif.: Synthesis Press, 1977), available only in libraries. See also Ram Dass and Paul Gorman's book, *How Can I Help?* (New York: Alfred A. Knopf, 1985), an elegant and touching study of the simplicity of service. People serve by moving in both directions: some of us heal ourselves by participating in healing the world, others focus on healing ourselves and, by doing so, participate in healing the world. "Let there be peace on earth, and let it begin with me." (Song title © by Jan-Lee Music, 1955, 1983, used with permission.)

   See *Still Here: Embracing Aging, Changing, Dying* (New York: Riverhead Books, 2000), Ram Dass' book written during his recovery from a stroke he suffered in 1997 at age 65. Dass writes about his surprise at finding peace in silence. He also wrote his experience of wisdom and ecstasy in mindfulness— experiencing the present moment.

8. "Forgiving is not forgetting; it's letting go of the hurt," says Mary McLeod Bethune in *Courage to Change* (New York: Al-Anon Family Group Headquarters, 1992). There isn't a lot of time for regret, self-pity, and playing the victim in this new paradigm. My past is part of what makes me who I am, and I am grateful for it. There is nothing more to forgive. Lewis B. Smedes, in *The Art of Forgiving: When You Need to Forgive and Don't Know How* (New York: Ballantine Books, 1997), suggests that forgiveness cannot be forced; we forgive when we are ready to be healed. He says that "forgiving is the only way to heal the wounds of a past we cannot change and cannot forget."

9. The Heartmates Foundation was formed in 2000 to broaden the scope of education and awareness for heartmates worldwide. You can read about its projects and purposes and make a gift when visiting the Heartmates Foundation page on the Heartmates Web site: <www.heartmates.com>.

Appendix A:
Self-Help Resources

Self-care is essential for recovery from the vicarious trauma you experienced with the onset of your mate's heart disease. Appendix A includes exercises to assist your healing. The first on relaxation applies to the body and mind.

The second exercise, the Evening Review, is a reflective exercise designed specifically to help you manage your personal boundaries. The review can also be used as a template for analyzing any behavioral pattern that you wish to explore or change.

The Partial Life Review, which follows, is a way for you to discover and reflect on your style and pattern of dealing with loss. Like the Evening Review, it can be used in preparation for making thoughtful decisions about changes that will facilitate your healing.

There is, finally, a family problem-solving model to guide you and your whole family to healthy solutions of the issues generated by heart disease. This model has six steps that you and your family can use when you have decisions to make or differences to resolve.

Relaxation

Relaxing your body and mind is crucial to recovery. Biofeedback, yoga, and meditation are practical self-care practices that offer you a healthy way to manage the stress of the cardiac crisis. Check local community education programs or your cardiac rehabilitation program for available classes.

The following exercise is provided to get you started. Requiring no more than ten minutes, it can easily be done anytime during your day. (Consider practicing it at the beginning or end of the day or whenever you take a break.) To maximize its effectiveness, do the exercise on a regular basis. Make it a priority in your daily routine.

You can practice this exercise on your own, with a friend, or with family members. Reading the exercise to yourself can be distracting, taking away from its effectiveness. Have someone else read the exercise to guide you (over time you will probably memorize the exercise). You can also record it. In either case, the reader should pause for a few seconds after each step, giving you time to follow the instructions.

Relaxation Exercise
Sit in a comfortable chair with your spine straight and your feet flat on the floor. Close your eyes and focus your attention on your breath. Follow its natural flow, in and out . . . in and out. . . . Take in clear, pure energy each time you inhale. Experience the release of tension as you exhale. . . . Don't change the pace of your breath in any way; your natural rhythm is perfect for you. Notice that with each breath you become more relaxed. . . .

Now focus on your body. Begin with your feet: first your right foot, then your left. Imagine all your tension flowing out through your toes and the bottoms of your feet. . . . Now allow the muscles in your calves and thighs to relax as well. First your right leg, now your left. Feel your legs warm and loose . . . feel how the muscles in your feet are relaxed. . . .

Now pay attention to your abdomen, where you may notice a distinct tightness. Let your breath fill your abdomen. . . . Exhale tension. . . . Now move your attention to your chest cavity, to where your heart is protected. Breathe in light to surround and fill your heart. . . . Feel the fullness, the freedom of release from worldly worries. . . .

Now focus on your back and your shoulders with their many muscles. Breathe energy into your back, your right shoulder, then your left. . . . Feel the tension loosen and slip from your body. . . . Feel your back and shoulders expand with the energy of the light. . . .

Now turn your focus to your arms and hands. First the right: Breathe pure energy into your upper arm, then the lower arm, and then into your hand. . . . Experience the tightness flowing out through your fingertips. . . . Now repeat, focusing on your left arm, hand, and fingers. . . .

Shift your focus to your neck and head. Feel your neck relax. . . . It gently holds your head above your body. Feel positive energy, the flow of light, run through it. . . . Concentrate now on your jaw, letting it relax, letting your mouth open naturally as you let go of holding it tight. . . . Now focus on your eyes; feel the muscles behind your eyes relaxing and expanding. . . . And last, be mindful of the top and back of your head. Feel your head get clear as the energy of light fills it. . . .

You are relaxed and alert. Your mind is no longer racing. You are safe and present in this moment. You are filled with a sense of peace and well-being.

Now imagine yourself in a beautiful green meadow. . . . You are at rest, being nurtured by the beauty surrounding you. You are held securely by the solid earth beneath you. Feel the warm sun and the gentle cool breeze on your skin. . . . The air is fresh. You smell wildflowers and freshly mown grass. You hear birds singing to each other. A butterfly flutters by in the distance. You enjoy the babble of a nearby brook.

Let the peace and calm of this moment wash over you. . . . Allow yourself to soak in the feeling of safety . . . of being still. Stay in this serene and beautiful place as long as you like and are comfortable. . . . When you are ready, focus your attention on your breathing again. Breathe fully and deeply. . . . Breathe in a quality you can use when you return to your world—serenity . . . patience . . . freedom . . . compassion . . . forgiveness . . . love . . . and exhale any remaining tension or tightness. . . .

Now very gently bring yourself and your awareness back to the present and slowly open your eyes. . . . Take a moment to look around and return your awareness to the room . . . then rise slowly. . . . As you rise, stretch your body tall, fingertips reaching for the sky. . . . Now, with your sense of peace and your new quality, step into your reality refreshed and strengthened.

Evening Review

The Evening Review is an exercise particularly useful to people in a health crisis because it provides a structure to establish regular introspection, a quiet time when you can think about your day. "Reviewing" can help you focus on vital questions raised by heart disease. Naturally operating during a crisis, "re-viewing" is a mental activity that helps to clarify reality, establish order in the midst of chaos, and structure a fresh perspective as you face uncertainty. It facilitates acceptance of reality in regular, small steps. The Evening Review, used daily, is a powerful recovery tool.

Evening Review Exercise

The Evening Review can be used to examine any particular aspect of your life, including inner processes or patterns you want to know more about. The exercise can be modified, too, to fit a specific need, as in the example on page 285, which applies to setting boundaries.

The attitude with which you approach your review is most important. When you examine your day, try to be a detached, objective observer, clearly registering what has happened without judgment or blame. Then move on to the next item of review without excitement, without elation at a success or disappointment about a failure. Aim for dispassionate awareness of your day. *Don't* relive it.

The review is best done as the last activity of your day. Before going to sleep, review your day going backward in time, "rewinding" it like a tape. Begin where you are right now, then observe evening, then the dinner hour, the afternoon, and so on backward through the morning to the moment you awoke.

Many people have found it valuable to write down observations, insights, or impressions as part of a journal or the Heartmates Assessment Diary (see page 71). Doing so helps them process their thoughts, feelings, and perceptions. Taking notes or journaling is also a tool for remaining objective. It will help you "get out" of the subjectivity of your feelings, allowing you to discover patterns and trends in your thinking and perceiving. This becomes especially true if you review your notes over time.

Remember that the review is intended to be an informational tool. It is not for rehashing feelings or criticizing your decisions or actions. It is a tool for awareness, clarity, and understanding. It can lead to empowerment, healing, and change. Keep your review simple and defined. Give it no more than fifteen minutes a day (including any writing), particularly during the first weeks you practice it.

Review of Boundaries
The Evening Review can be applied to any aspect of your life that you want to see more clearly. The following modification consists of reviewing your day from the point of view of your boundaries. Boundaries are protective "membranes," personal lines of defense, best used to attract that which nourishes and sustains you and to deflect that which does not. (Consider the plant that soaks up nutrients in appropriate quantities to sustain its growth.)

Before doing this review for the first time, identify activities and relationships that are particularly nourishing or depleting at this time in your life. Some additional things to keep in mind as a foundation for your Evening Review include:

- What is my experience of my boundaries? Have there been changes in my boundary system since the cardiac crisis began? Are there changes as I become aware of my boundaries and how I use them?
- How do I evaluate environmental influences? Which give me comfort and which do I need protection from?
- How skillful am I in using and shifting my boundaries? In what situations and with which people is it easy or difficult to be me?
- What do I allow in? What do I push away? What in myself do I protect (my heart, my mind, my body, my feelings)? [1]

You may consider these questions during the review itself, or you can consider them at the end of your review. They are meant to stimulate your thinking, to increase awareness about your boundaries and your needs as you heal from crisis. After a week or two of doing the boundary review, take time to revisit your notes, looking for patterns and trends. You can use what you learn from your reviews to make decisions about setting firmer boundaries where necessary and relaxing or modifying those that are too restrictive.

Focus on moving through your day, doing a short overview from the present moment back to when you awoke for the day. Divide the periods of the day by your activities. First take a mental snapshot of your evening. If you notice anything about boundaries, jot them down in your journal. Next look at the dinner hour. Ask yourself to notice your boundaries in relation to those with whom you prepared or ate dinner. Continue to go backward from the afternoon to the morning, getting a mental picture of the period with a focus on how your boundaries protected or didn't protect you during each activity.

When you are finished, set your journal aside. Do this for a minimum of a week before you reread your notes or try to distinguish a tendency or pattern.

Partial Life Review

People move through dark times into the light as they search for meaning. One of the natural ways people search is by reviewing what has happened to them in a crisis. This review is designed to help you analyze a transition or loss that you experienced prior to the cardiac event.

The exercise is particularly useful for identifying strengths and other qualities, developed in past crises, that you can apply and rely on now. Observe how you've handled loss in the past. Familiarize yourself with your unique patterns of coping. Your coping skills will expand as you see your strengths. You can incorporate the best of what you've done in the past with your newly developed skills and understanding.

You may want to do this review more than once, focusing on other life transitions. When you are familiar with your unique pattern of coping with transitions and loss, use the exercise to look at your present health crisis. Keep writing materials nearby. Insights, like dreams, are quickly forgotten unless they are recorded.

Partial Life Review Exercise

Take a few minutes to reflect on several events that were turning points in your life. Begin by jotting them down on paper. They might include a major decision you made, the loss of a relationship, or something that happened in society or in nature that had an impact on your life.[2]

Now, from those events you have written down, choose one that you are willing to look at in a more detailed way. Recall the period of your life when the event happened. What was going on within you, outside you? Who were the important people in your life? Did you confide in anyone? Were you alone, without support? As you review this period of your life, see yourself as you were then.

Now recall how you acted, what kinds of things you did when the event first occurred. Did you respond differently after the first few weeks? If you did, how so?

Notice your feelings about what was happening to you. Was there a progression of feelings as time passed, as you integrated the experience into your life? Did you express your feelings directly, or did you keep them to yourself and try to forget them? Did you express some feelings and suppress others? Did your feelings come out indirectly? Did anyone important to you know how you were feeling?

Now recall your thoughts at the time of the event. What were you aware of, considering, weighing, judging? Did you do that thinking alone or was there someone with whom you discussed those thoughts? At the time, did you ever think that what was happening was an opportunity? Did it make sense to you personally? How about in the larger context of your life, the life of your family, community?

Now, come back to the present, aware that that event was then and this is now. Does the event make sense in relation to your life now? Is there something you can see about it now that you couldn't see then? Does this review change in any way how you see yourself? Are you now more understanding, compassionate, accepting, and forgiving of what you did, how you felt, or what you thought of yourself then? Is there anything you learned then (a skill or a quality that you developed) that you can use now?

Is there anything in this review that points toward your future, any new way you'd like to act, live, think, or feel? Are there positive implications for the future, now that you have reviewed the past in this structured way?

When you have finished your review, take time to write about what you've learned. If it makes sense to continue the process, you may want to share your review with someone important in your life. You may want to continue your observation of this event, its implications, or the patterns revealed. Use the Evening Review for that purpose.

Family Meeting: Problem-Solving Guide

Families are vulnerable and unprepared when difficult decisions or long-term changes need to be made. Old conflicts erupt, complicating present concerns. Evolving roles and new family rules need to be clarified.

One method to deal with a health crisis as a family is to establish regular family meetings. Their purpose is to reestablish support and safety within the family, to discuss problems, and to seek solutions.

Family meetings should be scheduled weekly at a regular time and on the same day of the week. Take turns leading the meeting and sharing the responsibility of record-keeping (summary or minutes). Meetings should be no longer than one hour. Include family members of all ages. Children as young as elementary school age can participate. They will gain from being included, even if they have little to contribute at first (be sure to listen respectfully to contributions they do make).

The family will benefit if all members are willing to approach concerns as family issues, issues in which all have a part. The solutions to problems are as much a family responsibility as the problems themselves. This philosophy deepens mutual respect and cooperation and promotes family support and stability. The following is a six-step guide for seeking resolutions as a family:

1. Together, make a list of all the family concerns. The purpose of establishing this list is to define the issues and dilemmas

confronting the family. Anything unresolved in the eyes of even one family member belongs on this list. Be wary of commenting on contributions. This is not the time to share feelings about any perceived problems or concerns. Don't permit anyone to blame anyone else for any problem.

2. Together, select no more than three of the most critical issues. Selection should take into account which issues are the most urgent and critical to the family at the moment. Defer the remainder of the items on the list for later discussion. (Make sure the remaining items are introduced into "the record," the minutes for the meeting.)

3. Together, define what information is needed and which family members will be responsible for data collection. The goal of this step in the problem-solving process is to gather all the ideas, information, and outside resources that can help the family to resolve the issue. Family members can reflect on their ideas and feelings about each of the critical problems during the data-gathering period, then discuss their feelings at the following meeting. Set a realistic amount of time for data collection, and check on progress at the next weekly meeting.

4. Meet together to share information and resources. The purpose of this meeting is to share all the information and ideas on each of the critical issues to be resolved. Attentive listening and respect for each person's reflections are essential for success at this step.

5. Share individual ideas for solutions and resolutions. The most pressing problem should be discussed first, followed by the others in priority of importance. Designate one family member for each issue to be responsible for putting solutions in writing. Brainstorm solutions together. Important rules include: no interruptions, respectful listening, and consideration of every solution offered by all family members.

6. Agree on a best solution together. (Families reach agreement by consensus, negotiation, or compromise.) Then, decide

what actions will best accomplish your resolution and what each family member's responsibility is for carrying out those actions. Before taking on the next set of issues, schedule a follow-up meeting to ensure that your resolution on this issue is progressing or complete. Make sure to celebrate each solution as a family.

Appendix A Notes

1. Adapted from the unpublished writings of Roberto Assagioli.
2. Adapted from Rhoda F. Levin, "Life Review: A Natural Process," *Readings in Psychosynthesis: Theory, Process, and Practice* (Toronto: Ontario Institute for Studies in Education, 1985), 96.

Appendix B:
Heartmates Recommended Reading List

Consult the following list to read further about major topics discussed in this book. I have included some fictional and autobiographical works that I found inspiring as I worked on my recovery. Some of the books helped me with my feelings of loneliness and isolation.

Borysenko, Joan. *Fire in the Soul: A New Psychology of Spiritual Optimism*. New York: Warner Books, 1993.

———. *Pocketful of Miracles*. New York: Warner Books, 1994.

Boss, Pauline. *Ambiguous Loss: Learning to Live with Unresolved Grief*. Cambridge, Mass.: Harvard University Press, 1999.

Bozarth, Alla Renée, PhD. *Kinds of Loss*. Minneapolis: Compcare Publications, 1982.

Cameron, Julia . *The Artist's Way: A Spiritual Path to Higher Creativity*. New York: Tarcher/Putnam, 1992.

Carter, Rosalynn, with Susan K. Golant. *Helping Yourself Help Others: A Book for Caregivers*. New York: Times Books, Random House, 1994.

Courage to Change. New York: Al-Anon Family Group Headquarters, 1992.

Cousins, Norman. *The Healing Heart*. New York: W. W. Norton, 1983.

Dass, Ram. *Still Here: Embracing Aging, Changing, Dying*. New York: Riverhead Books, 2000.

Doerr, Harriet. *Stones for Ibarra*. New York: Penguin Books, 1978. This is a beautiful first novel by an elderly woman about a couple struggling to cope with a life-threatening illness.

Doherty, William J. *Intentional Family: Simple Rituals to Strengthen Family Ties*. New York: Avon, 1999.

Ericsson, Stephanie. *Companion through the Darkness: Inner Dialogues on Grief*. New York: HarperCollins, 1993.

Gray, John. *Men Are from Mars, Women Are from Venus: A Practical Guide for Improving Communication and Getting What You Want in Your Relationships*. New York: HarperCollins, 1992.

Frank, Arthur W. *At the Will of the Body*. Boston: Houghton Mifflin, 1991.

Herman, Judith, MD. *Trauma and Recovery*. New York: Basic Books, 1992.

Holt, Stephen, MD. *The Natural Way to a Healthy Heart: Lessons from Alternative and Conventional Medicine*. New York: M. Evans and Company, 1999.

Kabat-Zinn, Jon. *Full Catastrophe Living: Using the Wisdom of Your Body and Mind to Face Stress, Pain, and Illness*. New York: Dell, 1990.

Kenney, Susan. *Sailing.* New York: Viking Penguin, 1988. A novel about a middle-aged woman coping with losses, whose husband has cancer.

Kushner, Harold S. *When Bad Things Happen to Good People.* New York: Schocken Books, 1981.

L'Engle, Madeleine. *Two-Part Invention, The Story of a Marriage.* New York: Farrar, Straus & Giroux, 1988. An autobiography about the love of two very independent people sharing the last years of one partner's life.

Moore, Thomas. *Soul Mates: Honoring the Mysteries of Love and Relationship.* New York: HarperCollins, 1994.

Ornish, Dean, MD. *Love and Survival: The Scientific Basis for the Healing Power of Intimacy.* New York: HarperCollins, 1998.

Remen, Rachel Naomi, MD. *Kitchen Table Wisdom.* New York: Riverhead Books, 1996.

———. *My Grandfather's Blessings.* New York: Riverhead Books, 2000.

Seligman, Martin E. P. *Learned Optimism.* New York: Alfred A. Knopf, 1990.

Siegel, Bernie S., MD. *Love, Medicine & Miracles.* New York: Harper & Row, 1986.

Smedes, Lewis B. *The Art of Forgiving: When You Need to Forgive and Don't Know How.* New York: Ballantine Books, 1997.

Sotile, Wayne M. *Heart Illness and Intimacy: How Caring Relationships Aid Recovery.* Baltimore: Johns Hopkins University Press, 1992.

Strong, Maggie. *Mainstay: For the Well Spouse of the Chronically Ill.* Boston: Little, Brown, 1988.

Viorst, Judith. *Necessary Losses.* New York: Simon & Schuster, 1986.

Appendix C:
An Essay on Loneliness and Its Antidotes

Many heartmates decry their loneliness. Seldom do we understand how our mates' heart disease results in loneliness. We find ourselves dismayed, disappointed, and despairing. This excerpt from a letter illustrates the loneliness experienced by a forty-five-year-old heartmate:

> *My spouse has read* Heartmates, *too, and feels a greater understanding about the issues his illness has raised for me, for us, and for the family.* Heartmates *allowed him to step aside for a moment from his role as patient and be my friend again. It's been a hard and tender time of deep change.*

The question arises: how is it that what we want most, to feel loved and understood by our mates, is seemingly so difficult, so out of our reach, so impossible to grasp? The nature of heart disease and health-care offers some answers.

- Heartmates are given a strong message in the hospital (by our limited access to our mate and by the hush-hush atmosphere maintained in the coronary care unit) that the patient must be protected from stress. How we interpret the message, in our shock and terror, is that we—our presence and our very being—are dangerous to the patient. *We* could cause another cardiac event, even our loved one's death, if we don't behave appropriately.
- Many heartmates believe that feelings and thoughts may be contagious. Early in recovery we begin to conceal our negative thoughts and feelings, believing that we are protecting the patient and the rest of the family. We want to make sure they're not discouraged by the way we feel. Natural feelings like fear, sadness, disappointment, depression, and resentment, as well as realistic and practical concerns, become unacceptable topics for discussion.

- Family and friends expect heartmates to express gratitude for the patient's survival. Healthcare professionals expect us to be consistent cheerleaders and indefatigable caregivers for the patient. Outsiders think that because the patient survived and is physically recovering, everything has returned to normal. Because they've not had the experience, non-heartmates don't understand that *our lives are permanently changed.* They don't know we have losses to grieve and adjustments to make to integrate this new reality. They don't realize that there is no going back to a pre-heart-disease normal.
- Heart patients are absorbed in their own health and recovery. Their physical and psychic energies are consumed with their own healing and serious concerns about their survival. Most don't recognize the effects of their heart disease on others. For the heartmate, this is one of the deepest sources of loneliness.

Although neither mates, nor family and friends, nor even professionals always understand the effects of heart disease on heartmates, *our grief and feelings of loneliness are real.* To understand that your experience is normal takes hard-won self-acceptance. It takes guts to break through the wall of isolation separating you from those who have not fully understood you. It takes courage to risk rebuilding the heartmate relationship, to commit to caring again, when you might lose your love.

When we hear ourselves say, "This is too hard. It isn't worth the struggle. I can't do it," we must reach for the resources deep within ourselves. There we find qualities we never knew we had—faith, strength, resilience, indefatigability, perseverance, courage, and caring. Surely we won't let loneliness defeat us!

We have used our skills and strengths to give to others—to our recovering mates and our families. To deal with our own loneliness we must give to ourselves, build a relationship with our "selves." And we must ask for and receive what we need from others—to be heard, to be understood, to be accepted, and to be loved.

The antidotes to combating loneliness are steps to healing—your healing. They are simple in design but not always easy in practice.

1. Accept all of your thoughts and feelings. They are legitimate, natural, human. Nurture your relationship with the God or higher power of your understanding. The relationship between you and the divine is the only eternal relationship human beings can have.

2. Seek support from others: those trusted and loving people who can hear you without trying to fix you (heartmates aren't broken); those people who can accept what they hear as your thoughts and feelings, even if they are different from their own; those people who can listen with empathy, who can understand and feel compassion for you.

3. Express your thoughts and feelings with people who will witness your experience and listen without judgment. Heartmates need to tell and retell their stories, say how they felt and feel, and express their concerns.

Accepting our own thoughts and feelings and sharing them with others leads us to a new place, a place where we stand alone but are no longer lonely. We will know our uniqueness and our connection to others simultaneously. We will have our special place in the world and belong with all other humans. We will continue to heal the significant wounds of the cardiac crisis.

Stay connected. To network with other heartmates visit us on the Web at <www.heartmates.com> (see the "Interactive Connections" page there). To contact us, write to <heartmates@heartmates.com> or The Heartmates Interactive Connection, Box 16202, Minneapolis, MN 55416.

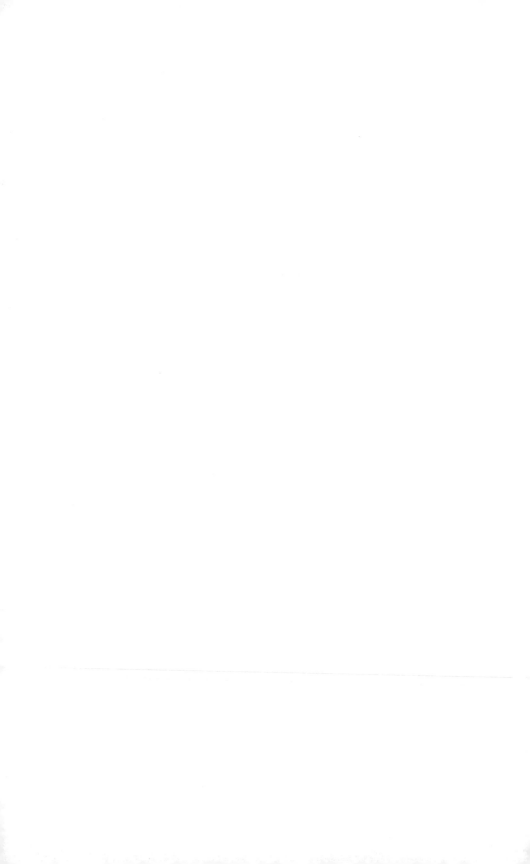

Appendix D:
An Essay on Stress

Stress can be defined as an automatic response your body makes to the demands placed on it. When a demand is made, adrenaline and cortisol are released and your body responds by going into the "fight or flight" pattern. When you need extra strength or stamina to fight or flee, adrenaline supplies it.

Stress exists both inside and outside of us. It affects us before birth and until we die. It affects us socially, spiritually, emotionally, psychologically, as well as physiologically.

The link between stress and illness is not so much about the illness, but our response to that illness. Having a partner with heart disease will cause a stress response. Family members are stressed by any situation that happens to one of their own.

Stress can be either positive or negative. Brief periods of stress, for example, are not necessarily harmful. When psychological stress accumulates and is not discharged (chronic stress), however, hormonal imbalances and lowered immune resistance may result. This puts us at risk because we are less able to fight illness.

Disease means the body is in "dis-ease," not at ease. Prolonged stress affects our bodies at their most vulnerable sites. Tension headaches and migraines, backaches, stomach pains, ulcers, and changes in the immune system have all been linked to prolonged stress.

Stress can be beneficial. Many people perform well under stress. A certain amount of stress helps us to concentrate, stay focused, perform, and even achieve peak efficiency. The key to coping with stress is to relax and enjoy the achievements, enabling the body to build for the next challenge.

Stress and its symptoms can be a wake-up call for the body to heal itself. When a situation, relationship, or illness is causing stress, we have the opportunity to examine the cause of the stress and make changes. Changing a behavioral or an emotional response may help physical, emotional, and spiritual healing. Stress management, then, has two components:

- understanding that stress is an inevitable, natural occurrence, and
- using the awareness of stress as an incentive to make positive changes in our lives.

In order to manage your stress, you must be aware of it. Learn what your stressors are and how stress affects you. Discover your emotions and learn to deal with them in a healthy way. Develop positive mental attitudes. Turn those attitudes into positive actions. Assess your problem-solving skills, and determine which you can develop further to ease the stress as part of your recovery.

Practice a regular exercise program. Exercise keeps your body in balance, increases stamina, and decreases your appetite. Maintain a healthy diet. Drink eight glasses of water every day.

Engage in relaxation exercises, meditation, massage, yoga, or biofeedback. Practice regularly. Any one of these will help calm your body and therefore your mind.

Develop spiritually. Studies demonstrate a positive relationship between prayer or religious observance and health. Religious or spiritual practice can be a comfort, reducing chronic stress.

Maintain a positive self-image. Recognize your needs and make healthy choices to support those needs. Decide to let go of grievances; learn to forgive and experience the freedom of no longer being a victim. Remember, there are few situations and no people, other than ourselves, that we can control.

Reach out to others for support. This is especially important to do when stress becomes unmanageable. Talk to trusted friends, family members, support groups, or a professional counselor. Talking with others, with those who will be there for you, will provide an important safety valve for your feelings of stress and reduce its future occurrence.

Learn to laugh—at yourself and with others. Studies have shown that laughter increases the immune response of the body. Always maintain a sense of hope. And last but not least, live in the present and look forward to the future.

Contributed by Pamela R. Borgmann, BA, RN, MTh, a massage therapist and founder of the Community Legacies Foundation.

Glossary of Medical Terms

aneurysm. A weakness in an artery or vein in the wall of your heart muscle that forms a balloon-like bulge.

angina. The heart muscle's complaint that it is not receiving enough blood or oxygen. It frequently occurs when the heart works harder than usual: during exercise, stress, sexual intercourse, a walk in extremely hot or cold weather, or after eating a large meal. Anginal discomfort can be experienced as chest pain, pressure, or heaviness. It can manifest as pain or aching in the jaw, teeth, or earlobes, or a choking or tightening sensation in the throat. It may be experienced as pain, aching, or numbness in one or both arms or hands, between the shoulder blades, or in the neck. Anginal discomfort may start in one place and move to another (i.e., chest pain that spreads to the shoulder and down the arm). It is important to understand that angina is not just "chest pain," but may be a variety of symptoms. Angina is usually brief, abating quickly or slowly from thirty seconds to five minutes. Angina is not a heart attack.

angiogram. A procedure that films the coronary arteries. A catheter (specialized tube) is inserted into an artery in the groin. It follows the artery's path up to the heart. Dye is injected through the tube while filming is done. These films show areas of narrowing or blockage in the coronary arteries and help the cardiovascular specialists plan the most effective treatment. This procedure takes about an hour and involves some risk, but it is one way to get a precise reading of coronary artery blockage. After the procedure, the patient must lie flat for several hours to prevent the artery from reopening and bleeding.

angioplasty. A procedure to increase blood flow to the heart muscle. A stent (a small wire-mesh tube) is placed in the coronary artery to hold it open. The stent is used in 70 to 90 percent of angioplasty procedures. A balloon angioplasty uses a balloon catheter (tube). When the catheter is positioned in the narrowed portion of the coronary artery, the balloon is inflated to compress the plaque. Widening the narrowed area of the passageway increases the flow of blood and oxygen to the heart muscle.

antiarrhythmics. A group of medications that regulate irregular heart rhythms.

anticoagulants (sometimes incorrectly referred to as blood thinners; they do not actually thin the blood). These medications are used to improve the flow of blood and prevent the formation of blood clots. (Blood clots blocking the coronary arteries can cause a heart attack.)

antihypertensives. Various medications used to lower high blood pressure.

aorta. The large main artery that leaves the heart to deliver freshly oxygenated
    blood to all parts of the body.

arrhythmia. Any change in the normal rhythm of the heart.

arteries. Blood vessels that carry oxygenated blood from the heart to all parts
    of the body. (Veins are the blood vessels that bring oxygen-depleted
    blood back to the heart.)

arteriosclerosis (also called hardening of the arteries). A progressive condition
    that causes the artery walls to thicken and lose their elasticity.

atherosclerosis. This is a form of arteriosclerosis, in which the passageways of
    the arteries become roughened and narrowed by fatty deposits that
    harden along the inner lining of the arteries. *See* plaque.

beta-blockers. A group of medications used to treat high blood pressure. Some
    beta-blockers are used to relieve angina and are taken to prevent addi-
    tional heart attacks. One side effect of beta-blockers may be impotence
    or reduced libido. Switching to a different beta-blocker may eliminate the
    side effect.

blood enzyme test. Cardiac enzymes are substances normally stored in the
    heart muscle. During an injury to the heart (a heart attack), these
    enzymes are released into the bloodstream. Blood samples are drawn
    after a suspected heart attack to check for these enzymes. This test helps
    to determine whether a heart attack has occurred. It usually takes
    twenty-four to forty-eight hours after the suspected heart attack to get
    results. *See* troponins.

blood pressure. The pressure placed on the walls of arteries by the heart
    pumping blood. The top number (systolic) refers to the pressure in
    arteries while the heart is contracting, and the bottom number (diastolic)
    refers to the arterial pressure when the heart is relaxed between beats.
    See hypertension.

bypass surgery (also called coronary artery bypass surgery, CAB, CABS). A
    blood vessel from another part of the body is used to bypass the blocked
    area in the coronary artery. The clean blood vessel is sewn above and
    below the blockage in the coronary artery. This construction provides a
    new pathway for blood to flow around the narrowed section of artery to
    the heart muscle. Imagine the surgery as providing a detour to avoid a
    traffic jam: the new pathway allows vehicles to get where they're going
    unimpeded. The procedure relieves angina for 90 percent of bypass
    patients and improves blood flow to the heart muscle.

calcium channel blockers. A group of medications used to treat angina by
    increasing the supply of blood and oxygen to the heart while reducing
    the work of the heart.

cardiac risk factors. These are lifestyle habits, physical attributes, and characteristics (inherited traits) that may increase the chance of developing heart
disease. Risk factors include smoking, high blood pressure, high blood
cholesterol, inactivity, obesity, diabetes, stress, and a family history of
heart disease.

cardiopulmonary resuscitation (CPR; also called mouth-to-mouth resuscitation). A lifesaving skill taught by the American Red Cross. All heartmates
should consider becoming CPR certified and renewing their certification
every three years. Preparation and training may help save a life. This skill
also builds confidence in the ability to respond appropriately and efficiently in an emergency.

cholesterol. A fatlike substance found in animal products (highest in organ
meats), dairy products, and eggs (highest in yolks). The cholesterol
present in the blood stream originates from cholesterol eaten plus that
produced naturally in the human body. Elevated blood cholesterol is
associated with an increased risk of hardening of the arteries. (*See* atherosclerosis.) There are several types of cholesterol. *See* fatty acids; lipoproteins; saturated fat; unsaturated fat.

cholesterol reducers. Medications that lower the level of cholesterol in the
blood. *See* statins.

congestive heart failure (CHF). A condition in which a weakened heart is not
able to pump blood adequately. Poor circulation causes fluid to collect in
the lungs, ankles, and feet.

coronary arteries. Three main arteries and their branches that supply the heart
muscle with blood, oxygen, and nutrients. If these arteries become narrowed, angina or a heart attack can occur.

diuretics. Medications that increase the output of urine, thereby helping to
reduce the amount of fluid and sodium retained in the body. They may
be used to treat high blood pressure and congestive heart failure.

echocardiogram (ECG). A way of viewing the heart without entering the body.
This technique uses high-frequency sound waves for measuring and
determining the function and structure of the heart. It is completely
painless and takes less than an hour to complete. Echocardiograms
cannot image coronary arteries at this time and, therefore, cannot be
used to pinpoint arterial narrowing. *See* angiogram.

electrocardiogram (EKG). A recording of the electrical currents produced by
the heart. These currents are responsible for the beating of the heart
muscle. A resting EKG can detect abnormal beats and determine if the
heart muscle is receiving enough blood and oxygen or if the heart has
sustained damage. This painless procedure involves attaching suction
cups (electrodes) to the skin.

endotracheal tube. Part of assisted breathing equipment, it is a tube that is placed in the windpipe. Endotracheal tubes are used during surgery, post-op, and with very ill patients. Bypass patients are frustrated and complain of this tube because they can't speak when it is in place. Having a pad and pencil, small erasable marker board, or Magic Slate available allows the patient to communicate until the tube is removed (usually twelve to twenty-four hours after surgery).

exercise. Forms of physical activity done by cardiac patients for the purposes of reducing risk factors, increasing physical fitness and quality of life, and possibly improving cardiac function. Studies show that walking, jogging, bicycling, swimming, and rowing (aerobic exercises) are activities that produce these results. It is generally recommended that people with heart disease engage in these activities three to five times a week for twenty to forty-five minutes. Check with your personal physician and cardiac rehabilitation center for specific guidelines.

fatty acids (also called trans fatty acids or hydrogenated fats). Found in the fats of the foods we eat, particularly in processed foods. Saturated fats, trans fatty acids, and cholesterol all raise blood cholesterol levels, a major risk factor for coronary artery disease. Studies show that trans fatty acids raise total blood cholesterol levels, but not as much as saturated fats. *See* cholesterol; lipoproteins; saturated fat; unsaturated fat.

gene therapy. Altering heart disease with gene therapy appears promising. Research includes stimulating new blood vessel growth (angiogenesis) and providing a built-in defense against blood clots that cause heart attacks.

heart attack (also called myocardial infarction, MI, or coronary thrombosis). Describes a condition when the flow of blood to a part of the heart muscle is suddenly and severely diminished or cut off entirely. The result is that a part of the heart muscle is damaged or dies.

homocysteine. An amino acid found in the blood that relates to heart disease and stroke risk. Research indicates that high homocysteine levels may damage the inner lining of arteries and promote blood clots. More conclusive studies are needed to establish a direct link to homocysteine and coronary artery disease.

hypertension (also called high blood pressure). Describes a condition when blood pressure is greater than 140 (systolic) over 90 (diastolic) in adults. High blood pressure is a cardiac and stroke risk factor. *See* blood pressure.

implantable cardioverter defibrillator (ICD). Used in patients at risk for ventricular tachycardia (rapid heart beat) or fibrillation (rapid, uncoordinated heart muscle movements). When an ICD detects ventricular tachycardia or fibrillation, it sends a shock to the heart, returning the heart to its normal rhythm.

lipoproteins (HDL, LDL). Fats carried in the blood, also known as "good cholesterol"(HDL) and "bad cholesterol"(LDL). Abnormal levels of these
fats are associated with heart and blood vessel disease. Triglycerides are
another type of fat found in the bloodstream. High triglyceride levels are
more commonly found in overweight or diabetic people who consume a
high-fat diet. *See* cholesterol; fatty acids; saturated fat; unsaturated fat.

nitrates. Medications commonly prescribed to treat angina. They increase the
supply of blood and oxygen to the heart while reducing the work of the
heart. They may be prescribed in several forms: a tablet to be dissolved
under the tongue (sublingual), a tablet to be swallowed (oral), or an oint-
ment or patch to be applied to the skin (transdermal).

nitroglycerin. A commonly prescribed, fast-acting medication used to treat
angina. *See* nitrates.

pacemaker. A mechanical implant that stimulates and regulates the heartbeat
by a series of regular electrical discharges.

plaque. In heart disease, plaque refers to a patchy deposit of fatty material consisting of cholesterol, calcium, and other materials, found on the inner
lining of coronary arteries.

post-cardiotomy syndrome (also called post-myocardial infarction syndrome
or Dressler's syndrome). A condition of inflammation in the sac covering the heart that may occur after a heart attack or heart surgery. It is
characterized by fever and chest pain (different from angina or incision
pain). It is treatable with anti-inflammatory medications such as aspirin
or cortisone.

saturated fat. A fat usually solid at room temperature. Common sources
include animal products (butter, chicken skin, marbled meats) and some
vegetable products (coconut oil, palm oil, cocoa butter, and hydrogenated vegetable oils). High dietary intake of saturated fats tends to elevate the level of cholesterol in the blood. Limiting foods high in
saturated fats may help to lower blood cholesterol. Studies and common
wisdom suggest that a heart-healthy diet limits fat to between 10 and 25
percent of caloric intake. *See* cholesterol; fatty acids; lipoproteins; unsaturated fat.

sodium. A mineral most commonly found in table salt. Sodium stimulates fluid
retention in the body, increasing blood pressure and making the heart
work harder. It is usually recommended that people with high blood
pressure or heart disease restrict sodium in their diet. Less than 2,000
milligrams is a sensible daily level to maintain. (There are high levels of
sodium in prepared and frozen foods.)

statins. A family of cholesterol-lowering medications that also reduce elevated
triglycerides and produce moderate increases in HDL cholesterol.

streptokinase (also called t-PA). A thrombolytic drug, enzyme, or substance
   that can dissolve blood clots. It is most effective when administered
   within one hour of onset of symptoms or within thirty minutes after
   arriving at an emergency room. If given immediately after a heart attack
   begins, it can help prevent heart muscle damage and reduce mortality by
   dissolving blockages in the arteries and restoring coronary artery flow.

stress test (also called a graded exercise test or GXT). This procedure tests how
   well the heart delivers oxygenated blood during physical exertion.
   Results are used to determine the level of fitness, to prescribe safe exercise levels, or to determine the presence of heart disease. There is no
   such thing as passing or failing the stress test. After being attached to an
   EKG machine, the person begins walking on a treadmill at a slow speed
   and incline. Both are gradually increased. Blood pressure and EKG readings are monitored by a professional for changes in blood pressure or
   heartbeats.

thallium stress test (also called a nuclear scanning, myocardial perfusion, blood
   flow, or imaging test). Usually done in conjunction with an exercise
   stress test on a treadmill or bicycle. A small amount of thallium is
   injected into the bloodstream during peak exercise. Pictures are taken
   immediately to determine the uptake of thallium in the heart muscle.
   This test shows how well blood flows to the heart muscle.

troponins. A cardiac muscle protein released into the bloodstream following
   heart muscle injury (a heart attack). Normally, troponin levels are very
   low. They increase significantly within four to six hours of cardiac
   muscle damage and can easily be measured with a blood test. *See* blood
   enzymes.

unsaturated fat. Includes polyunsaturated and monounsaturated fats, both of
   which tend to lower blood cholesterol. Major sources of polyunsaturated
   fats include a number of liquid vegetable oils: corn, sunflower, cotton-
   seed, safflower, and soybean. Monounsaturated fats are found in peanuts,
   peanut oil, olives, and olive oil. Fat should be limited to less than 25 percent of total daily caloric intake, with no more than one-third coming
   from each of the three types of fat: monounsaturated, polyunsaturated,
   and saturated. *See* cholesterol; fatty acids; lipoproteins; saturated fat.

vasodilators. Medications that dilate blood vessels to increase blood flow.

Updated 2002 by Vicki Shapiro, MS, CES, who has worked with cardiac
patients and their families in cardiac rehabilitation for twelve years.

Bibliography

Achterberg, Jeanne. *Imagery in Healing.* Boston: New Science Library, 1985.

Angelou, Maya. *On the Pulse of Morning.* New York: Random House, 1993.

Assagioli, Roberto. *The Act of Will.* New York: Viking Press, 1973.

_____. *Psychosynthesis: A Manual of Principles and Techniques.* New York: Penguin Books, 1965.

Bolen, Jean Shinoda, MD. *Goddesses in Every Woman.* New York: Harper & Row, 1984.

_____. *Goddesses in Older Women.* New York: HarperCollins, 2001.

_____. *The Tao of Psychology, Synchronicity and the Self.* San Francisco: Harper & Row, 1979.

Borysenko, Joan, PhD. *Fire in the Soul: A New Psychology of Spiritual Optimism.* New York: Warner Books, 1993.

Boss, Pauline. *Ambiguous Loss: Learning to Live with Unresolved Grief.* Cambridge, Mass.: Harvard University Press, 1999.

Boston Women's Health Book Collective. *Our Bodies, Ourselves.* New York: Simon & Schuster, 1971.

Bowman, Ted, MSW. *Loss of Dreams: A Special Kind of Grief.* 2111 Knapp Street, St. Paul, Minnesota 55108; phone or fax: (651) 645-6058.

Bozarth-Campbell, Alla. *Life Is Good-Bye, Life Is Hello: Grieving Well through All Kinds of Loss.* Minneapolis: Compcare Publications, 1982.

Brecher, Edward. *Love, Sex, and Aging.* Boston: Little, Brown, & Co., 1984.

Bridges, William. *Transitions: Making Sense of Life's Changes.* Reading, Mass.: Addison-Wesley Publishing, 1980.

Budnick, Herbert N., PhD, with Scott Robert Hays. *Heart to Heart: A Guide to the Psychological Aspects of Heart Disease.* Santa Fe, N.Mex.: HealthPress, 1991.

Cambre, Susan. *The Sensuous Heart.* Atlanta: Pritchett & Hull Associates, 1978.

Cameron, Julia. *The Artist's Way: A Spiritual Path to Higher Creativity.* New York: Tarcher, 1992.

Carter, Rosalynn, with Susan K. Golant. *Helping Yourself Help Others: A Book for Caregivers.* New York: Times Books, 1994.

Cousins, Norman. *Anatomy of an Illness.* New York: W. W. Norton, 1979.

_____. *Head First: The Biology of Hope.* New York: E. P. Dutton, 1989.

_____. *The Healing Heart.* New York: W. W. Norton, 1983.

Dass, Ram, and Paul Gorman. *How Can I Help?* New York: Alfred A. Knopf, 1985.

_____. *Still Here: Embracing Aging, Changing, Dying.* New York: Riverhead Books, 2000.

Davidson, Glen W. *Understanding Mourning: A Guide for Those Who Grieve.* Minneapolis: Augsburg Books, 1984.

Doerr, Harriet. *Stones for Ibarra.* New York: Penguin Books, 1978.

Doherty, William J., and Thomas Campbell. *Families and Health.* Newbury Park, Calif.: Sage, 1988.

_____. *Intentional Family: Simple Rituals to Strengthen Family Ties.* New York: Avon, 1999.

Dreikurs, Rudolf, MD, and Vicki Soltz. *Children: The Challenge.* New York: Hawthorn Books, 1964.

Eliot, Robert, MD. *Stress and the Major Cardiovascular Disorders.* Mt. Kisco, N.Y.: Futura Publishing, 1979.

Ericsson, Stephanie. *Companion through the Darkness: Inner Dialogues on Grief.* New York: HarperCollins, 1993.

Erikson, Erik H. *Vital Involvement in Old Age.* New York: W. W. Norton, 1986.

Ferrucci, Piero. *Inevitable Grace.* Los Angeles: J. P. Tarcher, 1990.

____. *What We May Be.* Los Angeles: J. P. Tarcher, 1982.

Firman, John, and James Vargiu. "Dimensions of Growth." *Synthesis* 3–4. Redwood City, Calif.: Synthesis Press, 1977.

Fossum, Merle A., and Marilyn J. Mason. *Facing Shame: Families in Recovery.* New York: W. W. Norton, 1986.

Fowler, James W. *Stages of Faith.* San Francisco: Harper & Row, 1981.

Frank, Arthur W. *At the Will of the Body: Reflections on Illness.* Boston: Houghton Mifflin, 1991.

Frankl, Viktor E., MD. *The Doctor and the Soul.* New York: Vintage, 1955.

Friedman, Meyer, MD, and Ray H. Rosenman, MD. *Type A Behavior and Your Heart.* New York: Fawcett Publications, 1974.

Gilligan, Carol. *In a Different Voice.* Cambridge, Mass.: Harvard University Press, 1982.

Gray, John, PhD. *Men Are from Mars, Women Are from Venus: A Practical Guide for Improving Communication and Getting What You Want in Your Relationships.* New York: HarperCollins, 1992.

Hackett, MD. "Men and Sex after a Heart Attack." *Harvard Heart Letter.* Vol. 11, no. 5. March 1986.

Halperin, Jonathan L., MD, and Richard Levine. *Bypass.* New York: Times Books, 1985.

Hays-Grieco, Mary. *The Kitchen Mystic: Spiritual Lessons Hidden in Everyday Life.* Center City, Minn.: Hazelden Books, 1992.

Hazelton, Lesley. *The Right to Feel Bad.* New York: Ballantine Books, 1984.

Heilbrun, Carolyn G. *The Last Gift of Time: Life beyond Sixty.* New York: Ballantine, 1998.

Helprin, Mark. *A Soldier of the Great War.* New York: Harcourt, 1991.

Herman, Judith, MD. *Trauma and Recovery.* New York: BasicBooks/Perseus, 1997.

Hoffman, Nancy Yanes. *Change of Heart: The Bypass Experience.* New York: Harcourt, Brace, Jovanovich, 1985.

Holt, Stephen, MD. *The Natural Way to a Healthy Heart: Lessons from Alternative and Conventional Medicine.* New York: M. Evans and Company, 1999.

John, Roger, and Peter McWilliams. *You Can't Afford the Luxury of a Negative Thought.* Los Angeles: Prelude Press, 1988.

Jung, Carl. *Memories, Dreams, Reflections.* New York: Vintage Books, 1965.

Kabat-Zinn, Jon. *Full Catastrophe Living: Using the Wisdom of Your Body and Mind to Face Stress, Pain, and Illness.* New York: Dell, 1990.

Kavanaugh, Robert E. *Facing Death.* Baltimore: Penguin Books, 1972.

Kenney, Susan. *Sailing.* New York: Viking Penguin, 1988.

Kopp, Sheldon. *Raise Your Right Hand against Fear, Extend the Other in Compassion.* New York: Ballantine Books, 1988.

Kübler-Ross, Elisabeth, MD. *On Death and Dying.* New York: Macmillan, 1969.

Kushner, Harold S. *When All You've Ever Wanted Isn't Enough: The Search for a Life That Matters.* New York: Simon & Schuster, 1986.

_____. *When Bad Things Happen to Good People.* New York: Schocken Books, 1981.

Larsen, Earnie. *Stage II Recovery: Life beyond Addiction.* Minneapolis: Winston Press, 1965.

Laurence, Margaret. *The Stone Angel.* Toronto: McClelland & Stewart, 1964.

Lear, Martha Weinman. *Heartsounds.* New York: Simon & Schuster, 1980.

L'Engle, Madeleine. *Two-Part Invention: The Story of a Marriage.* New York: Farrar, Straus & Giroux, 1988.

Leonard, Linda Scheirse. *The Wounded Woman.* Boulder, Colo.: Shambhala, 1983.

Lerner, Harriet Goldhor, PhD. *The Dance of Anger: A Woman's Guide to Changing the Patterns of Intimate Relationships.* New York: Harper & Row, 1986.

_____. *The Dance of Intimacy: A Woman's Guide to Courageous Acts of Change in Key Relationships.* New York: Harper & Row, 1989.

Lessing, Doris. *The Summer Before the Dark.* New York: Vintage Books, 1973.

Levin, Rhoda F. "Life Review: A Natural Process." *Readings in Psychosynthesis: Theory, Process, and Practice.* Toronto: Ontario Institute for Studies in Education, 1985.

Lewis, C. S. *A Grief Observed.* New York: Bantam Books, 1961.

_____. *The Four Loves.* New York: Harcourt, Brace, Jovanovich, 1960.

Lifton, Robert J., and Eric Olson. *Living and Dying.* New York: Bantam Books, 1984.

Lindemann, Erich, MD. *Beyond Grief: Studies in Crisis Intervention.* New York: Jason Aronson, 1979.

Luskin, Frederic, PhD. *Forgive for Good*. New York: HarperCollins, 2001.

Lynch, James J. *The Broken Heart: The Medical Consequences of Loneliness*. New York: Basic Books, 1977.

Maslow, Abraham H. *The Farther Reaches of Human Nature*. New York: Penguin Books, 1971.

McDaniel, Susan H., Jeri Hepworth, and William J. Doherty. *Medical Family Therapy*. New York: Basic Books, 1992.

McGoldrick, Monica, et al., eds. *Ethnicity and Family Theory*. New York: Guilford Press, 1996.

McGoldrick, Monica, Carol M. Anderson, and Froma Walsh, eds. *Women in Families: A Framework for Family Therapy*. New York: W. W. Norton, 1989.

Miller, Alice. *Thou Shalt Not Be Aware*. New York: New American Library, 1984.

Mitchell, Kenneth R., and Herbert Anderson. *All Our Losses/All Our Griefs*. Philadelphia: Westminster Press, 1983.

Moore, Thomas. *Soul Mates: Honoring the Mysteries of Love and Relationship*. New York: HarperCollins, 1994.

Moustakas, Clark E. *Loneliness and Love*. Englewood Cliffs, N.J.: Prentice-Hall, 1972.

Napier, Augustus Y., PhD, and Carl A. Whitaker, MD. *The Family Crucible*. New York: Bantam Books, 1978.

Needleman, Jacob. *The Heart of Philosophy*. New York: Bantam Books, 1982.

———. *A Sense of the Cosmos*. New York: E. P. Dutton, 1975.

Northrup, Christiane, MD, *Women's Bodies, Women's Wisdom: Creating Physical and Emotional Health and Healing*. New York: Bantam Books, 1994.

Ornish, Dean, MD. *Eat More, Weigh Less*. New York: HarperCollins, 1993.

———. *Love and Survival: The Scientific Basis for the Healing Power of Intimacy*. New York: HarperCollins, 1998.

———. *Program for Reversing Heart Disease*. New York: Random House, 1990.

———. *Stress, Diet, & Your Heart*. New York: Holt, Rinehart & Winston, 1982.

Paul, Stephen C. *Inneractions: Visions to Bring Your Inner and Outer Worlds into Harmony*. San Francisco: Harper, 1992.

Peck, M. Scott, MD. *The Road Less Traveled*. New York: Simon & Schuster, 1978.

Peele, Stanton, and Archie Brodsky. *Love and Addiction*. New York: New American Library, 1975.

Pincus, Lily. *Death and the Family*. New York: Random House, 1974.

Remen, Rachel Naomi, MD. *Kitchen Table Wisdom*. New York: Riverhead Books, 1996.

———. *My Grandfather's Blessings*. New York: Riverhead Books, 2000.

Rilke, Rainer Maria. *Letters of Rainer Maria Rilke, 1910–1926*. New York: W. W. Norton, 1969.

Rogers, Natalie. *Emerging Woman: A Decade of Midlife Transitions.* Point Reyes, Calif.: Personal Press, 1980.

Rubin, Lillian. *Intimate Strangers: Men and Women Together.* New York: Harper & Row, 1983.

_____. *Women of a Certain Age.* New York: Harper & Row, 1979.

Rubin, Theodore Isaac, MD. *The Angry Book.* New York: Macmillan, 1969.

Sarton, May. *Journal of a Solitude.* New York: W. W. Norton, 1973.

_____. *Kinds of Love.* New York: W. W. Norton, 1970.

Scarf, Maggie. *Intimate Partners: Patterns in Love and Marriage.* New York: Random House, 1987.

_____. *Intimate Worlds: Life inside the Family.* New York: Random House, 1995.

Scott-Maxwell, Florida. *The Measure of My Days.* New York: Penguin Books, 1979.

Seligman, Martin E. P., PhD. *Learned Optimism.* New York: Alfred A. Knopf, 1990.

Selye, Hans, MD. *The Stress of Life.* New York: McGraw-Hill, 1956.

Sheehy, Gail. *New Passages: Mapping Your Life across Time.* New York: Random House, 1995.

_____. *Passages.* New York: E. P. Dutton, 1976.

Sher, Gail. *One Continuous Mistake: Four Noble Truths for Writers.* New York: Arkana, 1999.

Shneidman, Edwin S. *Deaths of Man.* Baltimore: Penguin Books, 1973.

Siegal, Diana Laskin, et al., *The New Growing Older: Women Aging with Knowledge and Power.* New York: Touchstone Books, 1994.

Siegel, Bernie S., MD. *Love, Medicine & Miracles.* New York: Harper & Row, 1986.

Simonton, O. C., S. Simonton, and J. Creighton. *Getting Well Again.* Los Angeles: J. P. Tarcher, 1978.

Smedes, Lewis B. *The Art of Forgiving: When You Need to Forgive and Don't Know How.* New York: Ballantine Books, 1997.

Sotile, Wayne M., PhD. *Heart Illness and Intimacy: How Caring Relationships Aid Recovery.* Baltimore: Johns Hopkins University Press, 1992.

Speedling, Edward J. *Heart Attack: The Family Response at Home and in the Hospital.* New York: Tavistock Publications, 1982.

Stauffer, Edith R., PhD. *Unconditional Love and Forgiveness.* Burbank, Calif.: Triangle Publishers, 1987.

Stern, Ellen Sue. *Expecting Change.* New York: Poseidon Press, 1986.

Strommen, Merton P., and A. Irene. *Five Cries of Grief.* San Francisco: HarperSanFrancisco, 1993.

Strong, Maggie. *Mainstay: For the Well Spouse of the Chronically Ill.* Boston: Little, Brown, & Co., 1988.

Tatelbaum, Judy. *The Courage to Grieve.* New York: Perennial Library, 1980.

Tickle, Phyllis. *The Shaping of a Life: A Spiritual Landscape.* New York: Doubleday, 2001.

Veninga, Robert. *A Gift of Hope: How We Survive Our Tragedies.* Boston: Little, Brown, & Co., 1985.

Viorst, Judith. *Necessary Losses.* New York: Fawcett Gold Medal, 1986.

Waxberg, Joseph D., MD. *Bypass: A Doctor's Recovery from Open Heart Surgery.* New York: Appleton-Century-Crofts, 1981.

INDEX

A

A Soldier of the Great War, 196, 200
abandonment, fear of, 50, 52-53, 115-117, 120, 127-128, 135, 140, 148-151, 162, 179, 187, 206, 224-225, 235, 242, 265, 274
adapting, 33, 42, 44, 50, 68, 78, 100, 118, 137, 140, 155, 169, 185, 202, 205, 211, 219, 222, 251, 254, 259, 264, 290
adjustment, 25, 187, 218, 240, 248
advocacy, 61, 118. See also communication.
Al-Anon, 194, 279, 291
American Association of Cardiovascular and Pulmonary Rehabilitation, 85
American Heart Association, 77, 85, 218, 227
aneurysm, 299
Angelou, Maya, 169, 305
anger, acknowledging, 148-150; and blame, 63, 149; checklist, 62-63; in communication, 61-62, 190, 200, 207, 212; and disintegration, 148; and forgiveness, 160, 162-163, 222; as mask for fear, 24, 50-51, 58, 60, 63, 70, 76, 111, 127, 170, 192, 199, 207, 222, 242, 254; the ogre, 58, 61, 200; and release, 24, 61-62, 148-149, 191; usefulness of, 61, 63. See also feelings; grief; healing; pain.
angina, 28, 39, 217-218, 299-301, 303
angiogram, 3, 19, 93-94, 217, 299, 301
angioplasty, 3-4, 11, 13, 197, 217, 233, 256, 299
Angry Book, The, 226, 308
antiarrhythmics, 299
anticoagulants, 299
antihypertensives, 299

anxiety, and change, 36, 54-56, 58, 94; chronic, 52, 54, 190; and denial, 55, 189; the great paralyzer, 54, 57; numbness, 52; reducing, 30, 55, 83, 94, 172, 189, 199; symptoms of, 4, 52, 189; and travel, 36; and the unknown, 51. See also fear; feelings; sleep; uncertainty.
aorta, 300
appetite, 4, 35, 41-42, 187, 189, 298
appreciation, 7, 14, 18, 41, 44, 56, 74, 97, 111, 149, 159, 162, 178, 182-183, 196, 208-211, 218, 220-222, 225, 233, 235, 244-245, 250, 252, 257-258, 264, 272, 278; lack of, 24, 60
arguing, 24, 67, 148, 234
arrhythmia, 300
arteries, 5, 151, 299-304. See also coronary arteries.
arteriosclerosis, 300
Artist's Way, The, 104, 291, 305
atherosclerosis, 300-301

B

balloon angioplasty, 197, 299
beginning, new, 151, 167, 238, 272, 278
beliefs, 22, 25, 39, 44, 68, 73, 88-89, 92, 96, 103, 117, 135-136, 138, 179, 191, 205, 210, 253, 275. See also journaling; myth; spirituality; storytelling.
beta-blockers, 300
bickering. See arguing.
Bishop Clarkson Hospital, 134
blame, 23, 35, 63, 68, 82, 123, 127, 129, 133, 141, 149, 165, 201, 234, 247, 251, 265, 267, 284, 289

117, 144. See also family; feelings; helplessness; powerlessness; travel.

feelings, acknowledging, 49, 55, 82, 120, 148-150, 237, 266; assessment diary, 34, 69-72, 77-78, 93, 144, 211; covering up, 60, 67, 170; denial of, 130, 143; as energy drain, 27, 48-49, 65, 67, 121, 164, 167, 185, 187, 207, 270, 282-283; guidance with, 28, 100, 212, 257, 266; and hospital, 7, 9, 19-20, 47, 68, 99, 106, 174, 187, 242, 259; and lifestyle changes, 270; mistaken for stress, 17, 25, 48, 55, 119, 123, 125, 132, 164, 187, 198, 207, 212, 229, 236, 297-298; and pain, 49-51, 60, 66-67, 116, 127, 136, 138, 142, 147, 191, 251, 264, 266; of patient, 17, 35, 47, 50, 76, 99, 106, 113, 118, 123, 125-126, 130-131, 142, 170, 175, 184, 202, 206, 216, 219, 242, 247, 259-260, 293; releasing, 27, 141, 147-151, 191, 198, 207, 222, 247, 282; seeking support for, 47, 50, 59, 66, 95, 132, 146-147, 149, 164-165, 179, 194, 203, 247, 265; taking stock of, 34, 55, 69-72, 77-78, 93, 144, 211; trivializing, 66; wounds, 4, 21, 50, 141, 143, 162-164, 189. See also cardiackids; crisis; forgiveness; grief; helplessness; imagery; mourning; nightmares; responsibility; roles; self-help tools; spirituality; storytelling; stress; support; visualization; vulnerability.

finances, 29-30, 38, 54-55, 71, 109, 150, 160, 184, 203. 264. See also roles; work.

Fire in the Soul, 169, 275, 279, 291, 305

Firman, John, 279, 306

food, 17, 22-25, 41-42, 45, 88-90, 118, 136, 153, 164-165, 179-180, 277, 302-303; and change, 24-25, 50, 177; cheating, 25; efforts to please, 32;

issues, 25; as love, 24, 32, 233. See also cooking; diet; sodium.

forgiveness, 77, 141, 159-163, 222-223, 228, 277-279, 283, 288, 291, 298, 307, 309

Frankl, Viktor, 273, 278

friends, 4, 15, 17, 24, 31-35, 39, 43, 47, 49, 57, 62, 64, 66, 72-75, 81, 92-93, 97, 102-104, 106-107, 110, 112, 119, 121, 126, 133, 140, 142, 145, 157, 164-167, 177, 181, 183-186, 192-194, 199, 208, 212, 224, 228-229, 236, 240, 245, 247-248, 250-251, 258, 262, 270-272, 282, 293-294, 298. See also grief; leisure; support.

frustration, 8, 28, 35, 51, 53, 65, 72, 108, 118, 123, 127, 132, 153, 167, 170, 172, 182, 191, 193, 209, 238, 302. See also anger.

future, 3, 5, 18, 23, 28, 32, 51, 67, 72, 82, 88-89, 92, 99-100, 103, 107, 135-136, 140-141, 143, 150-151, 153-154, 158, 166-167, 210, 225-226, 258, 262-264, 268, 278, 288, 298

G

God. See spirituality.

Gray, John, 199, 291

grief, emotional support for, 164-165; five cries of grief, 168, 309; and loss, 64, 66, 77, 137-140, 168, 184, 191, 221, 238, 292, 294, 305, 307; physical support for, 164-165; spiritual support for, 165-166; stuck in, 140, 256, 265; suppression of, 140, 147. See also healing; myth; storytelling.

guilt, 23, 30, 33, 35, 45, 51, 60, 67-70, 76-77, 110, 134, 139, 156, 164, 181-182, 186, 191-193, 199, 207, 230, 232, 239, 247-248

About the Author

Rachael Freed, LICSW, LMFT, is a pioneer in family-centered care and the creator of the Heartmates resources, including *Heartmates: A Guide for the Spouse and Family of the Heart Patient* and *The Heartmates Journal: A Companion for Partners of People with Serious Illness*. Known internationally as an inspirational speaker, Rachael offers seminars for healthcare professionals and programs for cardiac couples. To inquire about a speaking engagement or workshop, email rachaelfreed@heartmates.com, or write to:

Rachael Freed
c/o Heartmates
P.O. Box 16202
Minneapolis, MN 55416

Rachael is also cofounder of The Legacy Center, which assists individuals in creating their spiritual-ethical will, and is the author of *Women's Lives, Women's Legacies: Passing Your Beliefs and Blessings to Future Generations*. She has five grandchildren: Sophie and Sam Stillman, and Mitch, Lily, and Harry Levin. Rachael lives in Minneapolis.